Midlife
Eating
Disorders

···

Your Journey
to Recovery

···

Cynthia M. Bulik, Ph.D.

DIRECTOR OF THE UNIVERSITY OF NORTH CAROLINA

CENTER OF EXCELLENCE FOR EATING DISORDERS

BLOOMSBURY

Praise for *Crave: Why* ....

"More than 7 million Americans struggle with binge eating disorder (BED), according to a recent Harvard-based study, yet few of us know much about the condition . . . Cynthia Bulik . . . helps shed light on the problem." —**Naomi Barr, O *Magazine***

"A must-read if you've ever struggled with out-of-control eating or the weight gain so often associated with binge eating disorder."
—**Aimee Liu, author of *Gaining: The Truth About Life After Eating Disorders***

"I applaud Dr. Bulik for tackling this complex subject in a practical, sensitive, and supportive way."
—**Tommy G. Thompson, former secretary of the Department of Health and Human Services**

"Dr. Bulik's no-nonsense, easy to read, respectful, and clear approach is refreshing. *Crave* helps us all better understand the illness while providing concrete tools and hope for a successful recovery."
—**Lynn S. Grefe, CEO of National Eating Disorders Association (www.nationaleatingdisorders.org)**

"*Crave* offers access to extraordinary clinical wisdom without the clinical distance."
—**Laura Collins, executive director of Families Empowered and Supporting Treatment of Eating Disorders (www.FEAST-ED.org)**

"Dr. Bulik empowers people who struggle with binge eating disorder to take action. She offers her incredible insight and knowledge of eating disorders with compassion and understanding in order to help people reach the ultimate goal: Success."
—**Kitty Westin, president of Eating Disorders Coalition for Research, Policy & Action**

Praise for *The Woman in the Mirror: How to Stop Confusing What You* Look *Like with Who You* Are

"Bulik has a life-changing message for women and delivers it well."
—*Library Journal*

"This compelling account of how feelings about our bodies affect us throughout our lives is filled with inspiration and hope."
**—Susan Ringwood, chief executive of beat,
the UK's leading charity supporting and
campaigning for people with eating disorders**

"An untethered look at the reality of how both our biology and environment contribute to devastating eating disorders and other problems with self-image. Brava!"
**—Chevese Turner, CEO, Binge Eating
Disorder Association (BEDA)**

Midlife Eating Disorders

Your Journey to Recovery

CYNTHIA M. BULIK, Ph.D.

Walker & Company
New York

Published by Walker Publishing Company, Inc., New York

A Division of Bloomsbury Publishing

All papers used by Walker & Company are natural, recyclable products made from wood grown in well-managed forests. The manufacturing processes conform to the environmental regulations of the country of origin.

LIBRARY OF CONGRESS CATALOGING-IN-PUBLICATION DATA HAS BEEN APPLIED FOR.

ISBN: 978-0-8027-1269-1

Visit Walker & Company's website at www.walkerbooks.com

First U.S. edition 2013

1   3   5   7   9   10   8   6   4   2

Typeset by Westchester Book Group
Printed in the U.S.A.

This book is dedicated to my patients. I have learned more from you than any book could ever teach me. Thanks for placing your trust in me and allowing me to accompany you on your recovery journeys. Your personal stories continue to enrich my understanding of these disorders, inform my research, and inspire me to work toward better understanding, prevention, and cure.

Contents

DISCLAIMER

All matters regarding your health require medical supervision. This book draws on my decades of experience as a psychologist and director of eating disorders treatment and research programs. It is neither intended nor designed to replace the opinions of your health care professional.

I have used my own clinical experience and have incorporated the personal stories of many patients, partners, and health care providers into this book. To protect their privacy, I have used pseudonyms and, in some cases, for clarity or caution, combined experiences or commentaries into one character. Some of the vignettes and quotes in this book may be disturbing, but they reflect the reality of midlife eating disorders. The take-home message remains that recovery or, at minimum, improved quality of life is possible at any age. There is hope.

Introduction:
Erase All Stereotypes

When someone says "eating disorder," what image do you conjure up? Chances are if you are like most people, you imagine a thin white upper-middle-class teenage girl. Surprisingly, you couldn't be more wrong. Whatever preconceived notions you may have about who suffers from eating disorders, it's time to erase them and start over. Granted, anorexia nervosa is more visible than other eating disorders; those afflicted are strikingly underweight, may look pale, and may have other signs of the disorder such as dry skin and brittle hair. Pictures of someone with anorexia are shocking and attention-grabbing. The media love anything with a provoking visual hook. That's why we are much more likely to read stories about anorexia in newspapers and magazines than stories about the less visual eating disorders such as bulimia nervosa or binge eating disorder (BED). Plus, people are more aware of the lethality of anorexia nervosa, and the media are always hot on the trail of any story about a celeb who dies, be it from anorexia nervosa, drug or alcohol abuse, or suicide. Most people are less aware that other eating disorders also carry a death toll. The landscape of eating disorders has changed and we have to update our understanding of what they are and who they afflict.

If we look at the numbers, the most common profile of someone with an eating disorder is a woman in her thirties or forties who struggles with weight control and suffers from BED. But countless women and men in midlife and beyond from all racial, ethnic, and socioeconomic backgrounds wake up each morning to an ongoing battle with eating and body image, with many suffering from anorexia nervosa, bulimia nervosa, purging disorder, BED, and night eating syndrome. Millions more lurk below the diagnostic radar with enough disordered eating to disrupt their lives, but not to receive an official diagnosis.

On the surface, eating disorders play out similarly in adults and teens, but the context and the impact on their own and their families' lives differs enormously. Some adults with eating and body-image-related disorders live productive lives and carry their illness around with them like a hidden secret. For others, eating disorders remove them from the playing field of life, impairing their ability to work, reproduce, and love.

In the medical field, typecasting eating disorders as teen disorders poses dangerous challenges for adult women and men seeking compassionate care. Primary care physicians, obgyns, and other health care providers may overlook these disorders in adults or, even worse, demean women for not having "grown out" of these adolescent problems or ridicule men for having a "girls' disorder."

Partners and children suffer when adult women and men are afflicted. The cost of treatment renders families destitute and destroys relationships. Intimacy is crushed by body image concerns. Trust in relationships is shattered as women and men desperately try to hide their illness from others.

The treatments that we currently use were developed primarily for adolescent girls. We are only now starting to tailor treatments to deal with the specific challenges faced by adult women and men: how to recover when you have to work, engaging partners in recovery, developing parenting skills, and protecting the next generation.

It feels as if the landscape has changed abruptly, and our understanding and compassion have lagged dangerously behind. This book will help adults understand "Why me?" and "Why now?" and guide them in designing their own recovery.

It will also give them renewed hope by identifying the best in evidence-informed age-appropriate care and resources available in the community for themselves, their loved ones, and their caregivers. It will help partners and family members understand these perplexing illnesses, develop compassion for those who suffer, and encourage self-care. Finally, it will help professionals appreciate the nuances associated with detecting and treating midlife eating disorders. After reading this book, the reader should not only have a better understanding of the causes and nature of adult disordered eating and renewed hope for recovery, but also be a confident health care consumer and be aware of developmentally appropriate resources available in the community for patients and caregivers.

The information in the book includes both facts and feelings. The scientific, medical, social, and psychological facts associated with eating disorders illustrate what we know. The feelings add a human face to the facts. We all know that individual experience is rarely the same as what we read in textbooks. Although each of our journeys is unique, by sharing stories and experiences, we can build empathy and understanding for those who suffer from eating disorders.

This book deals with all eating disorders. The constellation of factors that cause and maintain anorexia nervosa differs somewhat from those that cause and maintain BED. Yet bringing them together under one cover can improve understanding of how these disorders are similar and different. Personal stories inform our own journeys toward health and are a beacon of light for those grappling with recovery.

Part 1 lays out the facts covering the context of midlife eating disorders, clinical presentation of the illnesses, how they differ from eating disorders in youth, eating disorders in men, and the environmental and biological causes of eating disorders. Part 2 deals with some of the unique challenges faced by individuals with eating disorders in midlife such as relationships, pregnancy, and parenting. Part 3 speaks directly to individuals with eating disorders and gets at the heart of recovery. I lay out the types of treatment that are available, discuss how best to find compassionate care, and reveal my observations about the ingredients of successful recovery that I have compiled in working with individuals with all genres of eating disorders over the past three decades. Each chapter closes with a section called "Awareness and Action." Although not a self-help book per se, *Midlife Eating Disorders* goes beyond informing the reader of the facts about eating disorders in midlife by providing reinforcing activities that enhance awareness of the problems and provide a blueprint for actively initiating and maintaining recovery. These sections can also be used as valuable tools for providers to engage individuals in their care.

PART ONE

The Facts About Midlife Eating Disorders

CHAPTER 1

A Culture of Discontent: Why Midlife and Why Now?

Why midlife and why now? These are the first critical questions that we need to address before delving into the topic of disordered eating in adults. To do so, we need to understand the culture and context in which they occur. In part, I contend that the "Bigs" are to blame, those multibillion-dollar industries that have conspired to make us feel terrible about ourselves at any age. Big Diet, Big Cosmetics, and Big Fashion are mega-industries that have developed what is perhaps the most effective marketing strategy in the world. Coupled with the pervasive and global food and beverage disaster propagated by Big Food, Big Sugar, and Big Beverage, they have managed to trap us all in a culture of discontent.

There are several coordinated steps to their strategy that culminate in this discontent, and the various major industries are in cahoots. One profits from the discontent caused by another.

In the past, marketing strategies were more focused on what you own rather than who you are. The theme was based on keeping up with the Joneses by having the latest fashions or driving a flashy car. Although this approach is clearly still being used, an additional and more insidious strategy now dominates. This approach is more personal and targets not what you own, but the basic fabric of who you are and what you look like.

The essence of this new strategy is first to convince you that there is something fundamentally wrong with you. By planting a seed of discontent about some aspect of your appearance and then repeating that message over and over, the marketer causes you to gradually become dissatisfied with that feature. Some of the targets are the old faithfuls: gray hair, baldness, wrinkles, weight, and shape. But then they drill down with targeted mind worms: age spots, freckles, skin tone, size of your calves, color of your teeth, shape of your nails, size of your pupils, and the presence or absence of hair on your chest, your back, or your toes. A *New York Times* article reporting statistics from the American Association of Orthodontists revealed that the number of Americans eighteen and older getting braces or some other teeth-straightening treatment from an orthodontist jumped 58 percent between 1994 and 2010.[1] Translated, that means 1.1 million adults annually, up from 680,000. One marketing gimmick boiled down to a scenario in which a father takes his child to be fitted for braces only to have the orthodontist turn to the father and say, "What about you, Dad?" With the average bill for a course of braces running three thousand to seven thousand dollars, if Mom and Dad get braces, too, that could mean upward of twenty thousand dollars on teeth straightening—money that would be better invested in their child's college fund!

Once they have sown the seeds of discontent, the Bigs then intensify their efforts to persuade you that you can and "should" do something about your defect. They convince you that you are dissatisfied and that altering your defect would both improve your own quality of life and keep others from being exposed to your disturbing features; thus you become even stronger in your conviction to correct the perceived flaw.

In swoop the Bigs as the savior marketing the product, service, or surgery that will correct the defect they have convinced you that you have. They bolster the appeal by claiming that their solution will not only fix the problem but will also bring with it an absolute epiphany of happiness, contentment, and self-esteem. Convinced, you cave in and buy the product or service and may actually enjoy a fleeting uplifting experience—my toes no longer have hair, my age spots have faded, my abs look firmer—but the joy is ephemeral. And when the solution you paid for ultimately fails and your discontent returns, Big Food will help you binge your misery away and Big Pharma will help you medicate your discontent. The cycle continues, unabated, as the Bigs feed off one another's failures and profits.

Here's an outrageous example. "Outies are not in" was the leading line of a series of commercials that were designed to get you to go into the bathroom, lift up your shirt, and lend a critical eye to your belly button. As summer approached, the ads started propagating what amounted to belly button social anxiety disorder. "Afraid to show your belly button at the beach?" Olivia, age thirty-seven, found herself lifting up her shirt and wondering what it would be like to have a tidier, innie belly button. Next time she saw the ad, she read further. "Maybe umbilicoplasty is for you." She read further and saw that this was an outpatient procedure, requiring only light anesthesia; and the "after" pictures showed absolutely perfect belly buttons.

For a few thousand dollars and a little bit of recovery time, she could get relief from the newfound shame she was experiencing about her belly button. After saving up the five thousand dollars, she went ahead with the surgery. The advertised brief recovery period turned into a prolonged and painful postoperative infection that kept her from exercising for months. Olivia ate out of frustration, and her weight started to climb (Big Food supplied her with supersize portions of caloric-dense comfort food). That summer at the beach, she didn't experience a sense of pride about her newly crafted navel, because she was so horrified by her weight gain that she would wear only a loose one-piece bathing suit (enter Big Diet to offer her an array of quick diets to shed those pounds before summer's end). The next year, Olivia vacillated between periods of out-of-control binge eating and weeks of obsessively following the next popular diet craze. Her quest for a trendy innie paved the way for a continued cycle of disordered eating and dieting.

Jerry was reeled in by a different ad. At age fifty-five, he started to fret over his expanding love handles. He and his wife were having sex less frequently, and occasionally he had difficulty getting or holding an erection. Neither he nor his wife was too worried about it; they viewed it as a natural thing that happened to many aging couples. The hormones simply weren't raging quite as much as they used to. But then, while waiting to get a haircut, Jerry started reading a men's health magazine. An article was talking about not having to give up the old you, recounting miracle stories about men who had regained their youth with human growth hormone (HGH). He also noticed copious advertisements promising "daily performance." In the wall-size mirror of the salon's restroom, he grabbed his love handles, looked at himself, and decided he really didn't like what he saw. There's no reason to let myself go, he thought. I should try these products. They're available, so I owe it to myself and my wife to try them.

Jerry started taking HGH and got a prescription for a daily erectile dysfunction medication. He also started exercising—at first three times a week, but gradually increasing to daily and then twice a day. Although he liked the new sleeker look of his body, he wasn't satisfied and started focusing on his body fat percentage. He kept trying to get it lower and lower, and each time he reached a weight goal, he reset his sights on a new, lower goal. Jerry was quite pleased with his sexual appetite, but he failed to factor his wife's desires into the equation. While he was ready to rumba every day, her waning hormone levels didn't match his medically induced ones. She begged him to back off and found his preoccupation with his own body off-putting. She finally confronted him one day when she walked in on him naked on the scale. "You look sick!" she exclaimed. Seeing that he weighed only one hundred forty pounds at six feet tall made her realize that she had failed to recognize all of the warning signs, thinking that this was just another manifestation of a midlife crisis. The promises offered to Jerry by Big Pharma paved his way to years and years of turmoil battling an eating disorder.

Chevese Turner, CEO of the Binge Eating Disorder Association, emphasizes how the Bigs influence eating and weight. "Obesity and eating disorders are a capitalistic dream . . . we blame the individual instead of the food, diet, and pharma industries. We are on a merry-go-round that will be there for many kids for generations to come. Obesity and eating disorders are the result of the perfect storm of sixty-plus years of commercial diets and drugs that induced the rebound effect of weight cycling, plus the thin ideal of the 1960s, plus the inclusion of corn and sugar in everything we eat (not to mention growth hormones in meats). So all of this and much more have wreaked havoc on those predisposed to obesity and eating disorders. But instead of blaming industry for causing the problem, we blame the individual for having the problem. In fact, we create obesity prevention campaigns that blame and shame the obese individual so we can create some more eating disorders too! It's all about capitalism, consumerism, and keeping women slim and men buff!"

These stories are all relevant to adult disordered eating precisely because the Bigs have broadened their target to reach women and men of all ages. Teen girls and young adult women used to bear the brunt of the advertising "shoulds" when it came to appearance alterations, while older women were more commonly tantalized with recipes and gardening and older men with cars and lawn mowers; but the advertisers are keenly aware of two trends. First, the population is graying. Women and men over age forty-five comprise 34.4 percent of the U.S.

population.[2] Moreover, baby boomers are dogged in their efforts to retain their youthful vigor, and they have money to burn. Unlike teens, who have to ask their parents for cash, or young adults, who may still be paying off debts or just starting off on their own, older folks have deep pockets and in many cases will spare no expense to address the flaws highlighted by the Bigs.

The Bigs induced Olivia to spend five thousand on her navel and Jerry to spend thousands on his meds and gym membership, but we'll read in the following chapters that eating disorders are not simply reactions to toxic environments. In fact, genes, biology, personality, and culture are all factors. However, the toxic environments that are perpetuated by the Bigs play a considerable role in the demographic shifts we are seeing in eating disorders today.

AWARENESS AND ACTION

For this first awareness and action exercise, take a personal inventory of how Big Industry has affected you.

Look around at your house, your car, your reading material, your cosmetics, your personal products, and your medications and supplements and trace back to what led you to make those things part of your personal armamentarium. How many of the things that you own, belong to, or have undertaken were prompted by industry creating a sense of discontent that you then paid them to remedy? This list should NOT include things that you do for health, like gym memberships or pantries stocked with healthful foods, but only those products or services that purport to eliminate an externally imposed unhappiness.

Examples:

Target of discontent	Product
Lumpy midsection	Control-top hose
Balding	Shampoos and follicle stimulators for hair growth
Skin tone	Spray-on tan, tanning bed subscription, bleaching creams
Body hair	At-home waxing kits, laser hair removal
Discoloration of teeth	Whitening strips, dental whitening procedure
Under-eye bags	Eye serums, injectable wrinkle fillers, surgical eyelift
Varicose veins	Compression stockings, sclerotherapy, vein surgery
Cellulite	Creams and lotions, body wraps, liposuction

CHAPTER 2

Defining the Disorders: What Are These Eating and Feeding Disorders?

The diagnostic categories for eating disorders are not stable, and the boundaries are fuzzy. Although some people get one eating disorder and stay in that category for the duration of their illness, many cross over or migrate to different presentations over time. It's important to remember that diagnoses are descriptive. They give us a framework to understand someone's difficulties, and they are a way for providers to communicate efficiently with each other and be "on the same page." But everyone's eating disorder is unique. Eating disorders don't fit into nice little boxes.

Psychiatry likes to invent new mental illnesses with each new volume of their diagnostic bible, the *Diagnostic and Statistical Manual of Mental Disorders* (DSM). The revised DSM-5, to be published in 2013, will create a new landscape for eating disorders. To put things in context, DSM-I (published in 1952) was 130 pages long and included 106 diagnoses. DSM-II (1968) was 134 pages long and contained 182 diagnoses and DSM-III (1980) was 494 pages long and included 265 diagnoses. This particular version included anorexia nervosa and introduced "bulimia" to the world as a psychiatric diagnosis for the first time—although the term described a somewhat different syndrome than it does today. DSM-III-R (1987) was 567 pages and included 292 diagnoses. DSM-IV (1994) was 886 pages and contained 297 diagnoses. And now DSM-5 (changing from Roman numerals to the 5 to facilitate regular updates—5.1, 5.2, etc.) is on the horizon, and we will soon discover both how long this new tome will be and how many syndromes it will include.[1]

Diagnostic systems tend to create neat little categories, which people may think they need to fit precisely into in order to have a "real" disorder. This can lead people to think they don't have a serious problem, to view their problems as insignificant, to postpone treatment, and, worse yet, this kind of thinking can impede insurance companies from paying for treatment for disorders that fall outside of the diagnostic box. But unlike some areas of medicine, psychiatric disorders don't have clean laboratory tests to verify a diagnosis: There's no blood test for bulimia, and no X-ray can diagnose BED. These are clinical diagnoses, and most people who suffer from eating disorders are exceptions to the rule rather than textbook cases.

In fact, one of the motivating factors for the changes happening in DSM-5 is that so many people with eating disorders fell into the "other" category, which used to be called Eating Disorders Not Otherwise Specified (EDNOS). In some reports, 60 percent of people presenting for treatment did not have classic anorexia nervosa or bulimia nervosa, but rather fell into this catchall category.[2] A sure sign that something is wrong with your diagnostic system is when most people aren't captured by the categories.

The new diagnostic system is poised to do a few things in an attempt to rectify this shortcoming. The most impactful change is that BED will become a stand-alone diagnosis (more on that later.) Second, the system is positioned to add what are typically thought to be disorders of childhood—pica (eating nonfood substances), rumination disorder (repeated regurgitation of food that may be re-chewed, re-swallowed, or spit out), and avoidant/restrictive food intake disorder (lack of interest in eating or food, avoidance based on the sensory characteristics of food, or concern about aversive consequences of eating)—to form a combined Feeding and Eating Disorders category.

The DSM-5 committee is also aiming to make the flagship

diagnostic categories (i.e., anorexia nervosa, bulimia nervosa, and BED) more encompassing by broadening their criteria. This move alone would have reduced the size of the "other" category effectively; but, in a perplexing move, the committee added more disorders to the new "other" category, which they renamed Other Specified Feeding and Eating Disorders. This category is proposed to include atypical anorexia nervosa, subthreshold bulimia nervosa, subthreshold BED, purging disorder, and night eating syndrome. The establishment of this category could end up having the opposite effect by reinflating the size of the "other" category. The committee is even proposing what amounts to an "other other" category (i.e., Unspecified Feeding and Eating Disorder).[3] The world can fundamentally be divided into lumpers and splitters; the DSM-5 committee must have had an overrepresentation of splitters!

THE FUTURE OF SELECTIVE EATING DISORDER

Selective eating disorder, once just called picky eating, is the newest behavior pattern to come under consideration for "disordership." Some think that elevating picky eating to the status of a disorder is going one step too far. Dr. Nancy Zucker, director of the Duke Center for Eating Disorders, has valuable thoughts on the issue.[4] While not entirely ready to call selective eating a "disorder," Zucker is increasingly encountering adults whose food sensitivity is so severe that it affects their functioning. Her alarm bells started going off when she noticed that over 20 percent of the individuals presenting to her clinic were extremely picky eaters. This was not just the "I don't like Brussels sprouts" crowd, but people whose selective eating was interfering with their lives, their jobs, their relationships, and their parenting. Many adult selective eaters were deeply concerned that their picky eating was setting a bad example for their children. Says Zucker, "Eating is social. Family meals are the nexus of family communication, rituals, and teamwork. Selective eating can make such events a time of extreme stress for families who experience extreme aversion—and often fear—at the thought of eating novel foods."

Typically, the most avoided foods are fruits and vegetables, which raises concerns about the effect of selective eating on nutritional status and overall health. And this is not just about taste buds. Selective eaters may actually experience the look, the taste, or the feel of food differently than other people; or they may have had early negative associations such as stomach problems, choking, or acid reflux that may have changed the bodily experience and/or psychology of eating certain foods. To better understand this phenomenon, Zucker and collaborators at the University of Pittsburgh developed a national registry of picky eaters. Zucker thinks selective eating runs deeper than we understand and that these people are not only worthy of consideration for disorder status, but also deserve improved understanding and treatment. "What people don't get," she says, "is that picky eating can be absolutely crippling." She recalls one patient who would only eat plain bagels, chips, peanut butter, and cheese pizza (of a certain brand). Imagine the impact this had on his social life!

The primary disorders—anorexia nervosa, bulimia nervosa, and BED—as well as several of the "other" disorders do not differ by the age of the patient. The criteria for anorexia nervosa are the same for an eight-year-old as for an eighty-year-old. This is distressing to many, especially those who work with children, as the clinical presentations in children are even harder to put into neat boxes. For the purpose of midlife eating disorders, however, the following criteria are directly applicable.

One additional important note about eating disorder diagnoses is that they have been developed with women in mind. Sometimes this ends up being like trying to get a man to fit into women's clothes. We say the prevalence of eating disorders is lower in men, and for some of the eating disorders, this is probably true. But part of the gender imbalance might well be because the criteria we use to diagnose the disorders and the instruments we use to assess them were based on how the disorders manifest in women. For example, "I am satisfied with the size of my bust," is hardly a good screening question for body dissatisfaction in men.

Anorexia Nervosa

Anorexia nervosa is a perplexing and harrowing disorder. It comes in a variety of presentations and degrees of severity. Anorexia nervosa afflicts about 0.9 percent of women and 0.3 percent of men in the U.S. population.[5] Based on census numbers, this translates to about 1.1 million women and 340,000 men over the age of eighteen with anorexia nervosa in the United States. Anorexia nervosa afflicts individuals across racial and ethnic boundaries, although the prevalence is somewhat lower in African-American women,[6] suggesting the possibility of some protective mechanism—whether biological or sociocultural.

The DSM-5 criteria for anorexia nervosa will focus on "restriction of energy intake relative to requirements leading to significantly low body weight." The precise definition of low weight will consider age and sex, although a specific body mass index [BMI, or weight in pounds multiplied by 703, divided by height in inches squared (or weight in kg/height in m²)] will not be specified in the criteria. The criteria will include either "intense fear of weight gain" or an alternative that focuses less on fear and more on behaviors that interfere with weight gain (e.g., excessive exercise). The psychological component of anorexia nervosa will be earmarked in a manner similar to DSM-IV with a disturbance in how one's weight or shape is experienced, with undue influence of weight or shape on self-evaluation, or with the lack of recognition of the seriousness of low weight. There will continue to be two fundamental sub-types: restricting (i.e., no binge eating or purging) and binge-eating/purging as observed in the past three months.

There will be some important changes to the anorexia nervosa criteria in DSM-5. The good news is that the first criterion will no longer refer to a "refusal" to maintain body weight or "denial" of illness. This old phraseology, offensive to many, was paternalistic and pejorative and failed to account for the fact that anorexia nervosa—especially in later stages—tends to take on a life of its own, at times completely divorced from any drive for thinness, with patients struggling to be able to eat at all.[7]

DSM-5 may still waffle on what exactly is meant by low body weight. Three variations on language, namely "significantly low body weight," "significantly low weight," and "current low body weight," are all fairly nonspecific and provide little concrete guidance for the clinician. The good news is that amenorrhea (cessation of menstruation) will no longer be a required criterion. This change comes on the heels of a considerable body of research indicating that whether one continues menstruating or not has little bearing on how severe one's illness is. Women vary in the robustness of their menstrual cycles: Some continue menstruating despite severe emaciation, whereas others stop having their periods after they start restricting but before any appreciable weight loss.[8] Plus this criterion was meaningless for men and peri- and postmenopausal women.

Beyond the DSM. Aside from the official diagnostic criteria, there are many other hallmark features of anorexia nervosa, several of which appear to pre-date the onset of the eating disorder. A common cluster of traits includes:

* A paralyzing sense of perfectionism that often emerges prior to the eating disorder. For example, work may be

done and redone, with the quest for perfection ultimately
leading to incomplete tasks.

* Abysmally low self-esteem that is completely dispropor-
  tionate to the nature of the person. Individuals with
  anorexia may be exceptional at athletics and school, and
  adept socially, but they may selectively attend to only
  their "weaknesses," failing to acknowledge any positives.
  People with anorexia nervosa are often challenged to
  incorporate any positive perceptions of themselves into
  their self-concept.
* Extreme anxiety in childhood. Even if they were well
  compensated on the outside, on the inside, anxiety raged.
* Depression. While depression is another common trait, it
  does not universally pre-date the eating disorder.
* Extreme self-consciousness. Individuals with anorexia
  overemphasize the extent to which they are the subject of
  attention and may fear, for example, that others can see
  imperceptible changes in their weight or shape and will
  judge them accordingly.
* Preoccupation with symmetry and exactness. Individuals
  with anorexia might insist that things be lined up in order,
  or that books be cataloged by color, or they may spend
  time counting or rearranging and perfecting things in
  their environment.

Memory and cognitive functioning can also be compromised. Many people, especially when underweight, have difficulty with their memory, which often resolves once they are
re-nourished. A specific subgroup of people with anorexia has
been found to have deficits in other cognitive skills, such as set
shifting, or the ability to shift from one point of attention to
another. This may actually be a better marker of illness and be
found to exist both before the onset of the eating disorder and
after recovery.[9]

Body checking, defined as "frequent evaluation of one's body to gain information about size, shape, or weight," is another hallmark feature of anorexia nervosa.[10] You can body check in many ways, including repeatedly weighing, measuring, or pinching yourself, examining specific body parts in mirrors and windows, asking for others' opinions about your shape or size, comparing yourself to others, feeling for bones, and checking the fit of certain items of clothing. Although everyone may body check once in a while, people with anorexia nervosa often body check obsessively.

Other features associated with anorexia nervosa that do not elevate themselves to the level of diagnostic criteria are more related to the obsessive and compulsive features of the disorder. Many individuals with anorexia develop ritualistic eating habits, including extremely slow eating. Their food repertoire can also become extremely limited, or they may move food around on their plate, eat odd foods, consume an inordinate amount of condiments or non-nutritive sweeteners, chew ice, and drink large amounts of noncaloric beverages, all of which serve to further their eating disorder, decrease anxiety about eating, or provide a sense of fullness without consuming calories.

Living with Anorexia Nervosa: Susan. I should have died long ago. I am fifty, and I have had anorexia nervosa for thirty years. No one understands how my body keeps going. I am in pain every day, but I feel compelled to push through it. I have been in the hospital more times than I can remember; some of them I can't actually remember, which is quite terrifying. My brother has power of attorney because, when I get so severely ill, I simply cannot make intelligent decisions—my brain stops functioning. I am on disability because I have not been able to work for the past ten years. My nieces and nephews don't want to be around me; I scare them. It brings tears to my eyes that my own family refuses to hug me for fear that they might "break me" because of my fragile state. When I walk into a supermarket, I can feel people staring at me. I know I am emaciated. I can see my bones.

When I was younger, I thought I looked fat, but now I can see through my translucent skin, and I know that my arms look frightening. But when it comes to putting food on a spoon and putting it in my mouth, I just can't do it. The fear that comes up with eating is so intense that it completely overrides any sense of reason. I feel driven instead to put on my shoes and go outside for a walk—to burn off the few calories I ate during the day. Even just thinking about eating food frightens me.

THE PREVALENCE OF EATING DISORDERS IN THE UNITED KINGDOM

The 2007 Adult Psychiatric Morbidity Survey (APMS) conducted in the United Kingdom included a brief five-question screening for eating disorders called the SCOFF.[11] The SCOFF questions are:

* Do you make yourself Sick (throw up) because you feel uncomfortably full?
* Do you worry you have lost Control over how much you eat?
* Have you recently lost more than One stone [approximately fourteen pounds] in a three-month period?
* Do you believe yourself to be Fat when others say you are too thin?
* Would you say that Food dominates your life?

SCOFF copyright J. Hubert Lacey and John Morgan

The survey included an additional question, namely "Do your feelings about food interfere with your ability to work, meet personal responsibilities and/or enjoy a social life?"

Using the criteria of answering yes to two screening questions and also answering yes to the question about interference, the following percentages of women screened positive for eating disorders: ages 16–24 (5.4 percent); 25–34 (3.6 percent); 35–44 (2.5 percent); 45–54 (3.1 percent); 55–64 (0.9 percent); 65–74 (0.6 percent); 75 and older (0.1 percent). Overall 2.5 percent of British women screened positive for an eating disorder, which translates roughly into 550,000 women in the United Kingdom.

Bulimia Nervosa

The DSM-5 criteria for bulimia nervosa will not change dramatically from DSM-IV. In the United States, bulimia nervosa is somewhat more common than anorexia nervosa, occurring in about 1.5 percent of women and 0.5 percent of men.[12] For the threshold disorder, these numbers translate into 1.8 million women and 570,000 men with bulimia nervosa in the United States. If you look at the number of people who are one criterion short (sub-threshold conditions), those numbers go up substantially.

The hallmark features of the disorder are binge eating and compensatory behaviors. The DSM-5 criteria for bulimia nervosa will likely include the following features:

* Recurrent episodes of binge eating, defined as eating in a discrete period of time an amount of food that is definitely larger than most people would eat during a similar period of time and under similar circumstances coupled with a sense of loss of control over eating. It is the

experience of losing control over eating that distin-
guishes a binge from an episode of overeating.

* Recurrent inappropriate compensatory behaviors (e.g.,
self-induced vomiting, laxative use, excessive exercise).
* Duration and frequency on average once a week for three
months.
* Self-evaluation that is unduly influenced by body shape
and weight.

The diagnosis of bulimia nervosa will not be able to be
given if the behaviors occur only when someone is experiencing anorexia nervosa (i.e., then the appropriate diagnosis would
be anorexia nervosa, binge-eating/purging subtype). Bulimia
nervosa occurs in individuals who are of normal weight, overweight, or obese.

One notable change to the criteria in DSM-5 is the frequency with which an individual has to engage in binge eating
in order to receive a diagnosis of bulimia nervosa. In DSM-IV,
the criterion was twice per week for three months. Again,
guided by research, the new criterion is once a week for three
months. This change was motivated by the fact that individuals
who binge at this frequency do not differ significantly in any
meaningful way from individuals who binge twice per week.

An important question that the field has grappled with is
"Does size matter?" As written, the diagnostic criteria provide
little guidance for when is a binge a binge. Emphasizing the
out-of-control factor helps in defining the behavior, but intro-
duces another conundrum. Many individuals may feel like
they lose control when eating a normal amount of food. To
capture these differences, clinicians talk about "objective"
binge episodes (OBEs) in which the individual eats what would
truly be an objectively large amount by social comparison and
"subjective" binge episodes (SBEs) in which they feel out of
control when eating a normal or small amount of food. Granted,

the precise placement of the boundaries is fuzzy, and many hours have been spent trying to define when a binge is a binge, but the objective and subjective distinction is useful for patients, providers, and researchers.

Beyond the DSM. Like those with anorexia nervosa, individuals with bulimia nervosa commonly suffer from depression, anxiety, and low self-esteem. Perfectionism can also be part of the clinical picture, which can be complicated by the presence of impulsivity. Many people with bulimia will talk about a duality in their own personality that includes both introversion and a reactionary type of extraversion. One patient described it as being "a wallflower who likes to dance on tables." Embedded in these characteristics is a tendency to act without thinking, which can be associated with impulse control problems such as shoplifting, emotional lability (changeability), reckless spending, sexual impulsivity, self-harm behaviors, and alcohol and drug abuse. With its vacillating episodes of restriction and binge eating, concentration and memory can also be severely impaired in individuals with bulimia nervosa.

Living with Bulimia Nervosa: Raj. We told the children that my ulcer is the reason that I always leave the table to go to the bathroom after meals. My wife now knows about the bulimia, but she doesn't know what to do about it. I don't think she ever imagined the possibility that her husband could have bulimia nervosa. She has even come to the doctor's office with me when he refused to believe that a forty-year-old man could have an eating disorder. Every day at work, I eat two grande burritos for lunch, with a bag of chips and guacamole and a large energy drink, then go to the bathroom in the basement and purge it up. I have done this Monday through Friday for the past two years. At this point, I think it is just habit, but if I don't do it, I am completely beside myself and distracted for the rest of the day.

Sometimes, if I haven't done my lunch ritual, my urge to binge gets so intense in the evening. If my wife takes the kids somewhere, and I know I'm alone for a while, I can go through a box of cereal, a whole pizza, a container of ice cream, and whatever else I can find, and then get rid of it all before they come home. When the kids walk through the door jumping all over me, wanting to tell me about soccer practice or Bible study or whatever they were doing, I try to be excited with them. But my wife takes one look at my bloodshot eyes, and she knows what I have been doing while they were gone.

Binge Eating Disorder (BED)

The eating disorders section of DSM-5 includes a third official diagnosis, namely binge eating disorder. BED differs from bulimia nervosa by the absence of regular compensatory behaviors. BED used to be an orphan tucked away under the old EDNOS category, but DSM-5 intends to give BED its own listing for several reasons.

BED is the most common eating disorder, afflicting 3.5 percent of women and 2.0 percent of men in the United States.[13] This translates to 4.2 million women and 2.3 million men in the United States with BED. Since the publication of DSM-IV, an inordinate amount of research has gone into understanding the nature and treatment of BED. A voluminous literature has documented the presence of the disorder and the nature of co-occurring psychological and medical conditions, and many clinical trials have explored how best to treat BED with both psychotherapy and medications. With the inclusion of BED in DSM-5, many more individuals will qualify for treatment, which will also hopefully be covered by their insurance companies.

The essential features of the proposed DSM-5 criteria for BED include the following features:

* Recurrent episodes of binge eating defined fundamentally in the same manner as bulimia nervosa, but augmented by descriptors that characterize the speed of

eating, whether the person feels uncomfortably full, if the eating happens in the absence of hunger, or is associated with other negative emotions such as embarrassment, disgust, or guilt.

* The individual must experience distress over the binge eating.
* The frequency and duration is on average once a week for three months.
* Unlike bulimia nervosa, the individual must not engage in regular compensatory behaviors.

Changes to the BED criteria emerge from considerable research. Most notably, the criteria will be more in line with those for bulimia nervosa by focusing on binge episodes rather than binge days, as was the case in DSM-IV. In addition, both the frequency and duration criteria will change. Previously, binge eating twice a month for six months was the threshold requirement for a diagnosis of BED; that has been reduced, in parallel with bulimia nervosa, to once a week for three months. It is unclear why the committee has opted to keep the grab bag of descriptors of the nature of a binge when they are not included in the bulimia criteria. Both disorders center on the same behavioral phenomenon of binge eating, so it is unclear why we need this list in one diagnosis but not the other.

One potential consequence of reducing the frequency and duration criteria for BED would be the "opening of the floodgates," leading to an inordinate number of individuals being diagnosed with and seeking treatment for BED. Yet it appears that this is unlikely to be the case. Calculations indicate that the lifetime population prevalence will increase by only 0.1 percent, which would be unlikely to overburden the health care system—although it will require that additional providers be available should these individuals seek treatment.[14]

Beyond the DSM. The diagnostic criteria for BED do not include psychological features. Many argue that BED is as much a dieting disorder as it is a binge eating disorder and clarify that many people with BED develop cycles of binge eating and dieting in what can become a futile chase for permanent weight loss. Depression and substance abuse commonly co-occur.

Living with binge eating disorder: Donna. I remember as a child listening to my parents talk about missing food and my mom walking in on me after I baked cookies, asking me where they all had gone. I told her that I had burned them and had had to put them down the garbage disposal. Thus started a life of lies. I was teased about my weight during school and buried my pain in food. I have been binge eating since I was six, but I never knew what it was or that other people did it. As an adult, I would do the weekly grocery shopping for the family and not be able to wait to get into the car with the bags; I would eat cookies all the way home. I remember with shame having eaten my son's entire sixth birthday cake, all decked out in a Lego theme, before he and his friends got home from school for the party. I had to run to the store and buy a generic undecorated sheet cake just so they would have cake. I have never felt so ashamed. When the urges would come over me, nothing, not even disappointing my son, could stop me.

Avoidant/Restrictive Food Intake Disorder
Previously categorized as Feeding Disorder of Infancy or Early Childhood, this diagnosis has been proposed to be included in the eating disorders section of the DSM-5. This move was made in recognition of the fact that the symptoms of the disorder also occur in adults. This diagnosis includes people do not eat enough or show little interest in eating; those who limit their diet because of sensory features; and those who refuse food secondary to some aversive experience. The actual symptoms may include avoidance of eating, an inability to meet nutritional or energy needs, weight loss, nutritional deficiency,

having to rely on supplements or medical refeeding, and inter-ference with functioning. Since most of the information that we have on this syndrome comes from children, we expect that we will learn much more as more research attention turns to adults.

Purging Disorder and Night Eating Syndrome
Two disorders that did not receive official homes in DSM-5, but will be included in the Other Specified Feeding and Eating Disorder category, are purging disorder and night eating syn-drome. Disorders are placed in that category if there are not yet sufficient data to warrant their inclusion as bona fide diag-noses, but they are recommended for further study. As seen with the history of BED, this can be a stepping-stone toward becoming stand-alone disorders.

Purging disorder is an eating disorder variant in which the dominant behavior is purging. Individuals engage in purg-ing behavior in the absence of binge eating.[15] The DSM-5 crite-ria for purging disorder will focus on recurrent purging to influence shape and weight in the form of vomiting, laxatives, diuretics, or other medicines in the absence of binge eating. It will also include undue influence of weight or intense fear of gaining weight. Research to date suggests that purging disor-der can be particularly pernicious, as individuals may purge even after eating little or no food. Physical complications, in-cluding electrolyte imbalances, sores in the mouth and throat, and esophageal ruptures, can ensue. Like those with other eat-ing disorders, people with purging disorder commonly report anxiety and depression, as well as distress and impairment, associated with the illness.[16]

Living with purging disorder: Charlene. I got to the point where I just couldn't stand having food in my stomach. At first I only purged things that I thought might make me gain weight, like carbohydrates. It wasn't easy to purge in the beginning—something in my body resisted—but I kept at it until I could make the food come up. Sometimes I would purge three or four times to make sure I got rid of everything. If I was somewhere and couldn't find a toilet, I would panic about having the food stay in my stomach, frantically looking for somewhere to purge and getting more and more uncomfortable with the food inside of me. After about two years of purging, it didn't matter what I ate—I just had to get it out of my system. I didn't even need to put my fingers down my throat anymore; all I had to do was contract my stomach muscles and everything would come up. It got to the point where, even when I wanted to keep something down, I couldn't. I purged everything.

Despite a considerable body of literature, night eating syndrome will be included in DSM-5 only under the "other" category. First identified by Albert J. (Mickey) Stunkard in 1955, night eating syndrome was originally defined as comprising morning anorexia (i.e., no appetite), evening hyperphagia (i.e., consuming at least 25 percent of daily calories after the evening meal), and insomnia three or more times a week. Due to varying definitions, the prevalence of night eating syndrome has been estimated to be anywhere from 3 percent to 25 percent in community-based studies.[17] The DSM-5 criteria for night eating syndrome will include recurrent episodes of night eating, as manifested by eating after awakening from sleep or excessive food consumption after the evening meal. There has to be awareness and recall of the night eating and it cannot be better accounted for by external influences such as changes in the individual's sleep-wake cycle or by local social norms (e.g., dinnertime in Spain is often eleven P.M. or even midnight). The night eating has to be associated with significant distress and/or impairment in functioning.

    Living with Night Eating Syndrome: Erica. I'm a thirty-four-year-old married woman with two wonderful kids, working sixty to eighty hours per week in a high-powered position. On the outside, I appear to have my life completely together . . . but it's not. I'm constantly walking around with guilt, disgust, shame, and fear. Why? I have had night eating syndrome for the past six years, and it is crippling my life. I vividly recall the night it started. I had just gone through an "intervention" brought on by my husband because of my excessive exercise (I have a history of anorexia). When I woke up in the middle of the night, I was hungry. I recall thinking, "Hey, I should just eat . . . I'm obviously hungry, and I don't want to go back to anorexia." So I ate, just a bowl of cereal. That was the worst decision ever. That night started what I call "the cycle from hell"! Now, every night, sometimes two, four, six times per night, I wake up possessed by something that makes me feel like I have to eat to sleep. I feel like a drug addict! And it gets even worse during periods of high stress—deadlines at work, an argument with my husband. I just don't get it. During the day, I can barely look at food (probably because I ate all night), and I have complete control over what I eat. But at night, I feel no control . . . I'll literally eat peanut butter out of the jar, cake with my bare hands—all sweets and carbs that I usually don't really crave. The next morning, I feel groggy from the lack of sleep and hung over from the sugar high. I'll try to replenish the missing food so no one notices. I've tried locking cabinets and keeping the key outside in my car, tying my leg to my husband's, taking sleeping pills (which do make it worse), practicing relaxation techniques, hanging huge posters and signs saying GO BACK TO BED and STOP, eating plenty of healthy food during the day, drinking lots of water, taking leptin, 5-hydroxytryptophan, melatonin. I'm so frustrated because no one seems to know about this disorder, even doctors, making me feel like I'll never get better. I've gained fifteen pounds and am at the highest weight I've ever been . . . and the pounds keep coming! Oddly, people continue to shrug off my night eating and downplay the significance. You try waking up five or six times a night and see how that feels the next day . . . not good!

That covers the official landscape of eating disorders as proposed in DSM-5. The critical take-home message is that the vast majority of people with eating disorders are going to be some variation on the prototypes described here. Someone might have little bits of each of the disorders or experience different symptom clusters at different points of the illness. That is the norm. Just because someone doesn't fit a category perfectly does not mean there is not a problem. Just because someone doesn't fit perfectly in a category does not mean the eating disorder is any less severe or disabling. All of these behaviors can have severe effects on physical and mental health. In fact, many researchers and clinicians would love to get away from this preoccupation with diagnostic categories and move toward a complex dimensional way of thinking about eating disorders. The psychiatry world is not quite ready to embrace that kind of thinking, but it can be a helpful way to think about your own symptoms or those of someone you love.

One approach is to make a list of core dimensions associated with eating disorders—BMI, binge eating, purging, restricting, excessive exercise, shape and weight concerns, and night eating—and then evaluate the extent to which each of them characterizes your eating disorder. Oksana, who weighs ninety-eight pounds at five feet eight inches, runs five miles per day, and tries to eat fewer than seven hundred calories per day, could simply be labeled as having anorexia nervosa, restricting subtype, in the DSM-5 system. Dimensionally, however, she has problems on the BMI, restricting, shape and weight concern, and exercise dimensions, but no symptoms related to binge eating, purging, or night eating. In contrast, John, who weighs two hundred fifty pounds at five feet ten inches, binge eats twice a day for weeks on end, coupled with a week of fasting but no purging. He also awakens almost nightly and is unable to fall back asleep without eating. John has concerns in the BMI, binge eating, restricting, and night eating dimensions, but not purging, excessive exercise, or shape and weight concerns. This dimensional approach yields a matrix of symptoms, which could more effectively capture the broad range of presentations we see and also provide a clear focus for individualized treatment.

AWARENESS AND ACTION: WHAT IS NORMAL?

What is normal? On the surface, this is such a simple question, but in reality, it has occupied the great minds of philosophy, psychiatry, psychology, sociology, and other disciplines for eternity. The following two cases illustrate what is currently conceptualized as the line between a normal variant of human behavior and a disorder. The first case illustrates overeating, something we have all done at one time or another and a behavior that is not considered to be an eating disorder. The second case illustrates BED.

Overeating. Josh liked to eat. When he went home to his parents' house, his mother would still cook his favorite dishes even though he was well into his forties. His mother went all out to make sure the refrigerator and pantry were stocked with his favorite foods, and he would be met with freshly baked cookies, roast beef with mashed potatoes, creamed spinach, and pie! At dinner, she always offered seconds, and even though he was full, Josh didn't want to hurt her feelings, so he ate second helpings. He felt really overstuffed but decided to just take a run the next day and cut down a little. But then Josh woke up to her famous apple coffee cake, and he couldn't say no! That afternoon he went to the gym because he was feeling overloaded. That night at a family dinner, Josh ate healthy portion sizes and took seconds, but he had no room for dessert. He plopped down on the couch and spent the evening watching football with his father and uncle. He couldn't wait to get back to his own routine. Josh was overeating, but he was not out of control. He did not have an eating disorder.

Binge Eating Disorder. Lorenzo had always had a healthy appetite. When he was young, his grandmother always referred to him as "her best eater." When his schoolmates started teasing him about being overweight, his loving Italian grandmother continued to shower him with his favorite foods. Not one to turn down something tasty and not wanting to hurt his grandmother's feelings, he always obliged. Lorenzo managed to keep his weight under control throughout high school by joining the Ultimate Frisbee team. Yet even with regular training, he always seemed to have an extra layer of fat compared with the other guys. Once he hit college, Lorenzo stopped playing Ultimate, but he didn't stop eating, a pattern that continued well into adulthood. Now in his forties, he often waited until his wife and kids went upstairs for the evening, and he would eat alone in the kitchen—first, the leftovers from dinner, before moving onto bread with cream cheese, and then doughnuts or chocolate to finish with something sweet. He was disgusted with himself, but he couldn't stop eating, and this happened two or three times a week. One night, his wife went downstairs and found food and wrappers strewn across the kitchen table. Lorenzo was asleep amid the mess with his head on his arms. His eating was out of control. Lorenzo had BED.

Adapted with permission from *Abnormal Psychology*, 2nd ed. (Beidel, Bulik, and Stanley).[18]

Think about your eating patterns and those of people you might be concerned about. Have your or their behaviors crossed the line into a disorder? As you read the above vignettes, did you ever think, "Wow, that sounds like me!" and then question whether your eating was unhealthy? If you're not sure or if you're worried, the best course of action is to schedule an evaluation. Getting a professional opinion is the single best way to determine whether you have crossed the line from a normal variation on the theme into potentially dangerous territory. Putting your head in the sand and hoping things will just go away is unlikely to be effective. Once unhealthy patterns set in, they are more likely to progress to more serious problems rather than resolve spontaneously.

CHAPTER 3

What's Different About Midlife Eating Disorders?

Before we talk about what's distinctive about midlife eating disorders, it's important to acknowledge how they are similar to eating disorders that arise in adolescence or young adulthood. For most of the disorders, the clinical picture we see in midlife is strikingly similar to the one we see in adolescence. The presentation of anorexia nervosa has the same core features of low weight, drive for thinness, body distortion, and pervasive self-loathing of appearance. Moreover, the personality features of perfectionism and harm avoidance vary little across the life span. Family members and providers may encounter the same denial that anything is amiss and the hesitation to seek, if not complete avoidance of, treatment. A near phobic fear of food and fat fuel the illness, and the disorder terrorizes and paralyzes family members. Secrecy and partial information mar interpersonal relationships, and family members are challenged to comprehend what appears, on the outside, to be self-inflicted starvation. A pervasive sense of impotence plagues caregivers, and the sense of having your hands tied is even worse with adult patients because their privacy and autonomy are protected by law.

Bulimia also differs little in its core presentation across the age span. The same pattern of binge eating and purging, the same secrecy about compensatory behaviors, and the same shame about these behaviors occur at every age. Likewise, from what little we know, purging disorder takes the same form in adolescents and adults.

BED does seem to have some developmental differences, with the main ones being between childhood and the later years. In children, rather than calling it binge eating, clinicians and researchers refer to "loss-of-control eating." While patterns of uncontrolled eating occur, children are less able to quantify or label their eating episodes as binges. Older adolescents and adults, however, are able to appraise portion size and more clearly determine when an eating episode is out of control and constitutes a true binge, rather than an episode of overeating.

So, in terms of very basic clinical presentations, although much about the disorders remains the same across adolescence and midlife, some subtle differences do exist. The differences that emerge are related to context, comorbidity, and access.

Australian data also suggest that the prevalence of these eating disorders in adults is on the rise. Two studies separated by a ten-year period were carried out in South Australia. The 1995 study surveyed 3,001 individuals of a mean age of 43 and reported the following prevalences in women: 3.1 percent for binge eating, 0.7 percent for purging, and 1.6 percent for strict dieting or fasting. Ten years later, sampling 3,047 individuals with a mean age of 45.1, each of these estimates more than doubled, reaching 7.2 percent binge eating, 1.5 percent purging, and 4.6 percent strict dieting or fasting. The story was much the same for men (see chapter 4), meaning that the public health impact of these disorders is increasing.[1]

Clinical Presentation

One of the most perplexing features of anorexia nervosa to outside observers is that patients see themselves as overweight even when they are clearly emaciated. Often, loved ones simply have to "agree to disagree" and acknowledge that their perceptions of the patient's body size are vastly different. However, with midlife women in clinical settings, this distortion is not always evident. Some adult women and men will enter treatment acknowledging that they are underweight, though they remain as resolved as their younger counterparts in not wanting to change their size. Adult patients may say things like "I can see that my arms are skinny," or "I know that my collarbone and cheekbones make me look like I have cancer," suggesting that, at least with reference to some body parts, they are able to perceive their true body size. They may still experience some disconnect and see other parts of their bodies—typically their hips, waist, or thighs—as fat in comparison to those body parts they can accurately appraise.

Access

People in midlife can be at increased risk for any eating disorder simply because their stage of life affords them greater access to dangerous compounds that can be used in the service of weight loss. Whereas adolescents are still dependent on family for finances and, by virtue of living at home and being minors, have less privacy, adults have their own disposable income, can shop in person or online for purgatives, can create privacy situations that allow them to engage in uninterrupted disordered eating behavior, and can readily access dangerous Internet content that encourages disordered eating without parental controls. Adults can also leverage privacy laws to keep others from interfering with their eating disorder.

Very practical differences between adulthood and childhood make it easier for an eating disorder to go undetected. An adult can drive to a grocery store, get food in a drive-through, binge in the car, be alone at home after work or work alone at home, go on a business trip—all of which can conceal disordered eating behavior. Coupled with the fact that eating disorders aren't on the midlife radar screen, people might observe suspicious patterns and even wonder about them but, because they are unsuspecting, never put two and two together.

A pharmacist won't look twice if a woman or man in midlife or beyond purchases ipecac, laxatives, diuretics, or diet pills. They could be for the customer's grandchild or ailing parents, or for use in their job as a visiting nurse. If a teenager attempted to purchase any of those, eyebrows would (hopefully) rise. That, of course, is because the pharmacist stereotypes eating disorders as an adolescent problem. An adult can go online and use a credit card to purchase any number of unregulated weight loss products, whereas additional hurdles exist for adolescents who do not yet have their own means of making Internet purchases. Adults can join several gyms and drive from one to another to engage in excessive exercise, whereas adolescents may not have the disposable cash for gym memberships and often need to be chauffeured by their parents.

Finally, if adolescents lie about their eating behavior, parents can parent. They may search rooms or cars, check browser history, punish children for untruths, restrict access to high-risk activities, remove children from school, and even commit them for treatment. Parents can take control of the situation. If an adult with an eating disorder lies to her or his spouse or partner, although that becomes a serious issue for the relationship, the partner can't parent. Adult patients can simply leave home, skip town, separate, or divorce, all because of the liberties afforded by adulthood. Although psychiatric commitment is possible, it occurs in only the most severe cases. Far more cases result in destroyed relationships before they ever reach that point.

Drugs and Alcohol
In clinical settings, we have seen a greater number of patients in midlife whose health picture is complicated by alcohol or drug abuse. Although adolescents have been purchasing alcohol illegally for decades, the legal drinking age is an important barrier to access. Adults with eating disorders may find themselves drinking instead of eating. Although the term "drunkorexia" was coined for the college population who starve all day

to "save up" calories for their evening drinking binges, adults with eating disorders may drink to stave off hunger pangs or to give them some pleasure in a life otherwise deprived of reinforcement. Adults with BED may alternate between—or even combine—food and alcohol binges. As alcohol is known to disinhibit restrained eating and also stimulate appetite briefly,[2] many adults find that drinking alcohol can trigger a binge. If both issues aren't addressed in treatment, a relapse in one area can easily trigger a relapse in the other.

Jasmine was first treated for alcohol abuse when she was seventeen years old. She entered rehab and recalled basically trading booze for cookies and diet cola. She and many other patients would walk around carrying two-liter bottles of caffeinated diet soft drinks like they were security blankets, desperately grasping for something to help manage their urges to drink. Her alcohol cravings were quickly replaced by intense sugar cravings, which started as midnight kitchen raids and progressed to all-out binges and purges before she even left rehab. During that first hospitalization, Jasmine got over her alcohol problem but left with bulimia. As long as she wasn't drinking, the staff seemed to think they had done their job. Over the next three years, she continued to binge and purge, sometimes at an alarming rate. She stayed sober, but the twenty-five extra pounds she was carrying around were too high a price to pay. She kept having to buy new clothes, and she felt puffy, tired, and ashamed. Jasmine tried to diet, but her body rebelled against the hunger. She felt deprived and desperate and reasoned that one drink would take the edge off her hunger. Well, Jasmine couldn't have just one drink and she quickly slipped back into her old patterns of alcohol abuse. To gain control, she was forced to go back into rehab, but the treatment center didn't seem to know what to do about her eating disorder. She binged and purged throughout her thirty-day stay, and the counselors simply recommended that she get treatment for her bulimia once she was discharged. At no point did any provider recognize the critical importance of treating both the alcoholism and the eating disorder at the same time.

We have also noticed many midlife adults with eating disorders who report both licit and illicit drug abuse. Pamela's relationship was built on evenings spent smoking marijuana with her fiancé, Tim. It had been part of their life together since college and was a comfortable pattern they had developed. The pair enjoyed spending time together, getting high, and then making love afterward. This pattern seemed to calm Tim and helped him sleep at night. Unfortunately, it did not have the same soothing effect on Pamela. As she would watch Tim peacefully fall asleep, she developed powerful cases of the munchies night after night. This progressed into frank binges, with their habit of smoking together fueling her eating disorder. Unsure what they would have left to share without their smoking ritual, Pamela was hesitant to divulge her shameful secret to Tim, who was blissfully unaware that she was doing anything but sleeping comfortably beside him.

This scenario is not uncommon, especially as many baby boomers who grew up with access to marijuana continue to incorporate it into their otherwise typical lifestyle. However, some might find that the effects it has on them as they mature differ from the effects they recall from when they were young.

Adults are also quite adept at extracting prescriptions from their physicians. If an eating disorder is not on physicians' checklists for midlife patients, they may be unaware that the medications they are providing are feeding directly into eating pathology. Adult women have reported success at getting prescriptions for thyroid conditions, attention deficit disorder, high blood pressure, and diabetes, even when they had no medical indication for these drugs, all of which the women were actually taking to help them lose weight.

Pain medications can also be abused by adults with eating disorders. Adults with BED report more chronic pain conditions than otherwise healthy individuals,[3] although it is not the only eating disorder in which pain is an issue. The medical consequences of long-standing eating disorders can lead to considerable pain throughout the body. Dental pain, gastrointestinal pain, and musculoskeletal pain can all lead individuals to seek a variety of pain medications to deal with the secondary long-term effects of anorexia or bulimia nervosa. The abuse of prescription medication can complicate both the clinical picture and the treatment of eating disorders. It can also influence motivation for treatment, as well as its effectiveness.

Jason had been suffering from severe bulimia since he was fifteen years old. Now thirty-five, he had destroyed most of his teeth from repeated vomiting and had severe dental pain. In addition, a herniated cervical disk from a biking accident had left him with residual neck pain, which was especially excruciating when he vomited. He also started feeling numbness down his arms after particularly vigorous bouts of self-induced vomiting. Jason's dentist prescribed acetaminophen with codeine, and his primary care physician started him on a low dose of oxycodone, which was gradually increased as it became less and less effective at controlling his pain. The medication caused constipation, so he reverted to his old habit of laxatives to counteract that side effect. Jason was locked in a vicious cycle of pain, bulimia, opiates, and laxatives.

Decades of suffering from an eating disorder wears down the body. While younger patients seem to defy biology and find ways to will themselves into continuing activities of daily living despite low body weight or frequent purging, many older patients find the same struggle increasingly difficult to maintain. They may turn to a variety of medications to increase energy, decrease pain, and help them sleep—to the point where they completely lose their native biological capacity to self-regulate. Recovery from the eating disorder also means dealing with these drug dependencies, which can be an even greater deterrent to treatment. Not only are they unwilling to relinquish the symptoms of the eating disorder, but the fear of giving up the drugs creates worry that they will no longer be even minimally functional in life.

Medical Problems

Eating disorders affect a range of bodily symptoms, and their effects differ by both disorder and severity. Individuals in midlife may be more vulnerable to physical problems simply because their bodies are older and less resilient. Women and men who have suffered from eating disorders for a long period of time place enormous physical demands on their bodies as they starve, binge, use laxatives, purge, exercise excessively, and engage in other behaviors associated with their disorder. The table on page 44 lists the most common medical problems associated with anorexia nervosa, bulimia nervosa, and BED.

Expanding on the table, anorexia nervosa in midlife can be particularly damaging to the gastrointestinal and musculo-skeletal systems. Years of anorexia or anorexia coupled with normal aging can lead to serious GI distress, gastroesophageal reflux disorder (GERD), constipation, and even pancreatitis. Osteoporosis becomes a serious concern as bone thinning associated with aging is exacerbated by starvation.

Adults with bulimia nervosa commonly report physical symptoms such as fatigue, lethargy, bloating, and gastrointestinal problems. The disorder is hard on the body. Frequent vomiting leads to erosion of dental enamel, swelling of the parotid (salivary) glands, and calluses on the backs of the hands (Russell's sign). Those who frequently misuse laxatives can have edema (bodily swelling), fluid loss and subsequent dehydration, electrolyte abnormalities, serious metabolic problems, and permanent loss of normal bowel function.[5]

Both men and women with BED report reduced quality of life because of health issues.[6] Some, but not all, of the complications associated with BED are secondary to obesity, such as Type 2 diabetes, gallstones, high blood pressure, stroke, digestive

PHYSICAL SIGNS AND SYMPTOMS ASSOCIATED WITH EATING DISORDERS

Adapted from Nuray Kanbur and Debra Katzman, "Physical Signs and Symptoms Associated with Eating Disorders" in *Restoring Our Bodies, Reclaiming Our Lives*, ed. Aimee Liu. (Boston & London: Trumpeter, 2011).[4]

Bodily system	Anorexia nervosa	Bulimia nervosa	Binge eating disorder
General and psychological	Weight loss or lack of weight gain Feeling cold Dehydration Fatigue Irritability and mood changes Depression Anxiety	Weight fluctuations Irritability and mood changes Dehydration Fatigue Substance use problems	Weight gain Weight fluctuations Mood changes Depression Anxiety Insomnia and sleep problems Pain Alcohol use
Head, eyes, ears, nose, and throat	Dry, cracked lips and tongue Parotid gland swelling (if purging)	Dry, cracked lips and tongue Palatal scratches Sore throat Sores in mouth and throat Painful teeth and gums Tooth decay or cavities Dental enamel erosion Parotid gland swelling (if purging)	Gum infections Tooth decay
Cardiovascular	Dizziness Chest pain Abnormal heartbeat (too fast, too slow, irregular) Very slow heart rate (bradycardia) Postural hypotension (rapid drop in blood pressure when going from lying or sitting to standing) Cold or blue hands or feet Poor circulation Ankle swelling Heart failure Sudden cardiac death	Dizziness Chest pain Abnormal heartbeat (too fast, too slow, irregular) Very slow heart rate (bradycardia) Postural hypotension (rapid drop in blood pressure when going from lying or sitting to standing) Ankle swelling	Shortness of breath Chest pain Stroke High blood pressure

Bodily system	Anorexia nervosa	Bulimia nervosa	Binge eating disorder
Pulmonary	Aspiration (entry of foreign material in lungs, if purging) Pneumonia	Aspiration (entry of foreign material in lungs, if purging) Pneumonia	Pauses in breathing during sleep (sleep apnea)
Gastrointestinal	Feeling full sooner than normal or after eating less than usual Episodes of abdominal pain and discomfort Constipation Bloating after meals	Heartburn Blood in vomitus Mid-upper-belly tenderness Diarrhea or constipation Peptic ulcers Pancreatitis	Heartburn Digestive problems Feeling uncomfortably full after eating Gallbladder disease
Metabolic	Chemical/electrolyte (salts in the blood and body fluid) imbalance in the body that affects the heart and other major organ functions	Chemical/electrolyte (salts in the blood and body fluid) imbalance in the body that affects the heart and other major organ functions	High cholesterol
Renal (kidney)	Frequent urination Kidney stones		
Endocrine	Absent menses Bone fractures Delay in the onset of pubertal development Growth delay	Absent or irregular menses	Irregularities in blood sugar Type 2 diabetes
Dermatologic	Dry skin Pale color to the skin Fine downy hair (lanugo) on the cheeks, upper arms, chest, thighs, back Brittle nails Yellow or orange discoloration of skin (carotenodermia) Thin, dry, brittle hair	Calluses on the back of the hand (Russell's sign) Dry mouth	Excessive sweating

Bodily system	Anorexia nervosa	Bulimia nervosa	Binge eating disorder
Musculoskeletal	Fatigue, muscle weakness, cramps Osteopenia and osteoporosis	Fatigue, muscle weakness, cramps	Decreased mobility Joint and muscle pain Osteoarthritis
Neurological	Decreased concentration, memory, thinking ability Peripheral nerve damage Structural brain changes	Decreased concentration, memory, thinking ability	Difficulty sleeping and poor sleeping habits Headache
Reproductive	Infertility Birth complications Babies small for their gestational age	Infertility Birth complications Hyperemesis	Infertility Birth complications Babies large for their gestational age Cesarean section

problems, and high cholesterol. We know very little about the long-term effects of BED that starts in childhood. Longitudinal studies are being started now that will help us understand the impact of long-term exposure to binge eating on health.

Psychological Problems

As mentioned previously, eating disorders often do not travel alone, and midlife is no exception. Two of the most common psychological companions are depression and anxiety. The association between eating disorders and mood disorders has been widely documented, with between 20 percent and 83 percent of individuals with eating disorders also suffering from depression. About one third of individuals report that the depression started before the eating disorder, while the remainder report either that the depression started around the same time or that the eating disorder came first.[7] Depression can live on even after the eating disorder is remitted; and women with eating disorders are also at increased risk for postpartum depression.[8]

Anxiety disorders also go hand in hand with eating disorders, with over 55 percent of individuals with anorexia and 68 percent of individuals with bulimia nervosa reporting having at least one anxiety disorder.[9] Unlike depression, more patients recall the anxiety disorder existing before the eating disorder, often as early as childhood.[10] Anxiety disorders take many forms in people with eating disorders, including more generalized forms of anxiety (e.g., anxious or worrying about a number of things), social anxiety, panic disorder, post-traumatic stress disorder, and obsessive-compulsive disorder.[11] People with BED who also have social anxiety report even greater concerns about their shape and weight regardless their BMI.[12]

Given that anxiety is so pervasive in individuals with eating disorders, and that it often pre-dates the eating problem, we see anxiety as one critical pathway into eating disorders. Many of the behaviors that make most of us more anxious (such as dieting, being hungry, vomiting) are experienced as anxiety-reducing by individuals with eating disorders. People with anorexia nervosa report that food restriction decreases their innate sense of anxiety, and individuals with purging disorder, bulimia, and BED report that engaging in disordered eating behaviors, be they binge eating or purging, calms their anxiety, albeit temporarily.

Outcome
How do individuals with midlife eating disorders fare in the long run? The data are definitely not complete, but the outcome of eating disorders does vary somewhat by type. Recovery is discussed extensively in Part 3. Again, it is important to remember that all of these statistics are complicated by the fact that eating disorder categories are fluid and that people commonly migrate across diagnoses. Recovery statistics from anorexia nervosa are not terribly encouraging, with full recovery in around 46.9 percent of patients, improvement in 33.5 percent, and a chronic course developing in 20.8 percent of whose who survive the disorder.[13]

Evaluating outcome across more than five thousand patients in different studies, close to 45 percent of patients with bulimia nervosa showed full recovery, whereas 27 percent improved considerably and nearly 23 percent had a chronic course. We do not know whether the outcome of midlife bulimia differs from statistics derived from adolescent or young adult cases. When age is considered, the data are mixed, with some studies suggesting that older age is associated with better, worse, or similar outcome.[14] In short, we just don't know.

Because BED is a recent addition to the DSM, we know less about long-term outcomes. In one study, six years after treatment, 57.4 percent of women had a good outcome, 35.3 percent an intermediate outcome, and 5.9 percent a poor outcome.[15] From the sample of sixty-eight, one patient had died, 6 percent still had BED, 7.4 percent had developed bulimia nervosa, and 7.4 percent continued to have some form of EDNOS. With an average duration of 14.4 years, BED can be a chronic illness, suggesting that is not just a temporary condition.[16]

Self-harm, Mortality, and Suicide

Eating disorders can be lethal. Many people are surprised to discover that anorexia nervosa has the highest mortality rate of any psychiatric disorder, estimated to be 5 percent per decade of follow-up.[17] People with anorexia nervosa are 10.5 times more likely to die than their age- and sex-matched peers.[18] Approximately half of the deaths result from physical complications of the disorder, such as malnourishment or heart failure, whereas the second leading cause of death in anorexia is suicide.[19] For this reason, friends and family members always need to take anorexia nervosa seriously. Thinking that it is "just a phase" or that someone will "snap out of it" risks losing that person forever. The best estimates we have that combine data from a number of studies suggest that individuals with bulimia have 1.93 times the mortality risk compared to a reference population.[20] Again, we know less about BED.

Self-harm also occurs in those with eating disorders. Self-harm can include cutting, burning, pinching, and other behaviors that are engaged in to achieve a sense of release. Self-harm is another symptom that many find difficult to understand. Placed in the context of the eating disorder, many core eating disorder symptoms involve pain, although these are generally not considered to be forms of self-harm. Starvation, binge eating, purging, cramping and diarrhea from laxative abuse, and excessive exercise are all pain-inducing behaviors. Another form of self-harm seen in individuals with eating disorders is rage that is taken out on the body. Examples include punching the stomach for being perceived to be too large, or pinching and grabbing body parts out of disgust or despair about being too fat. Scratches and bruises can reflect the deep self-hatred that these individuals feel in their darkest moments.

Suicide among those with eating disorders is a serious concern, underscoring the gravity of the illnesses and the critical importance of receiving adequate care. Combining data across several studies encompassing more than 16,000 patients revealed that individuals with anorexia nervosa are more than 30 times more likely to die by suicide than comparable healthy people in the population.[21] The same approach with more than 1,700 patients with bulimia generated an estimate of 7.5 times greater likelihood of death by suicide. The same study observed no suicides in individuals with BED with an average follow up of around five years.

We studied more than eight million people throughout Sweden and found that 1.6 percent of men and 2.0% of women overall reported suicide attempts. In contrast, 10 percent of men and 15 percent of women with anorexia nervosa reported suicide attempts. This translates into men and women with anorexia being almost eight and nine times more likely to attempt suicide, respectively, than their peers in the general population.[22]

Collateral Damage

When Alita was ill, she firmly believed that her two boys never noticed anything was wrong with her. She would cook meals and sit with the family, but then just pick at her food. She tried to put on a good show. Occasionally, she would disappear for a week or two when her weight dropped to a dangerous low, as she would have to be admitted to the hospital for refeeding. Invariably, she would leave against medical advice and return home weighing a little more, but far from well. Looking back years later, when she had fully recovered, Alita realized there had been a lot of "collateral damage." Her oldest son revealed to her that, even though he was young at the time, during every stay in the hospital, he feared she would never come back. Alita's anorexia had completely blinded her to the impact her absences had on her young sons and her husband. In retrospect, she labeled anorexia as "the most selfish of disorders."

When an eating disorder strikes an adolescent, aside from the patient, the next most affected people are the parents. In fact, caretaking for anorexia nervosa is as challenging for parents as taking care of someone with schizophrenia.[23] Siblings also suffer. An eating disorder can demand enormous time and effort from the parents, both when the patient is ill and during the treatment process; and that process often involves active parental and sometimes family engagement. Siblings can feel short-changed, or as if all attention—good or bad—goes toward the ill sibling. Finances are disproportionally directed toward the ill sibling, which can influence not only day-to-day needs, but also major decisions such as college choices. Figure 1 illustrates who in the family tree is most affected when the patient is an adolescent, while Figure 2 paints a strikingly different picture and illustrates the collateral damage Alita mentioned when she reflected on the impact her disorder had on her family.

In these figures, circles stand for females and squares

Impact of Adolescent Eating Disorder

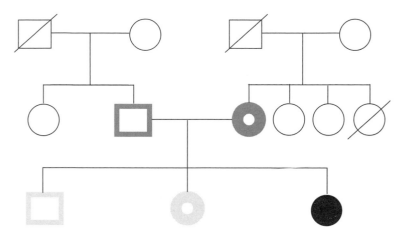

stand for males. A line through either symbol indicates that the person is deceased. A line connecting two symbols from the middle indicates a union. In Figure 1 (above), you can see that the adolescent daughter is affected with an eating disorder. The biggest effect is on her parents, as indicated by the thick, dark shading. Her sister and brother are also affected, but to a lesser extent than her parents. Her mother's sisters and her father's sister are not at all involved, and the parents have not even informed the living grandmothers about what is happening with their daughter.

Figure 2 (next page) presents a very different story. In this case, the affected individual is the mother, who finds herself right in the middle of her family of origin and her own family. Her husband is clearly affected by her eating disorder, as are her three children, especially the girls. In fact, one of them has started showing signs of disordered eating herself. The patient's two sisters are also affected, as they have been called in to baby-sit the children when the patient is in the hospital, and they are also deeply worried about their sister's health because the

Impact of Adult Eating Disorder

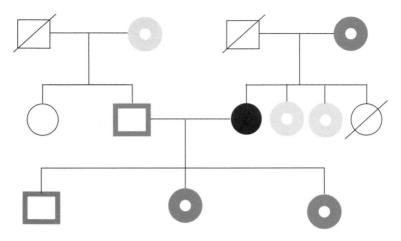

three of them have always been incredibly close. The patient's mother is not only worried about her daughter (and now grand-daughter) but is also affected because her three daughters have less time to spend with her since so much time is dedicated to caring for the patient and her children. Even the patient's mother-in-law is affected, as she, too, has been called in to babysit and cook for the kids on occasion when the patient is faring particularly poorly. So Figure 2 illustrates just how far-reaching the impact of an eating disorder can be when an adult is affected—and this is just within the family.

Impact on Friendships
Eating disorders in adults can induce extreme feelings of isolation and build thick walls between the sufferer and her or his closest friends. On the most practical level, people with eating disorders avoid eating with other people. Lunches at work, dinner with another couple, and parties where food is served all become "no-go zones" for the person with an eating disorder. Friends will extend invitations only so many times before assuming that further attempts are futile.

More subtle patterns can also emerge. Some individuals with eating disorders will continue to eat out with others, but it is a painful experience—both for the sufferer and for everyone else at the table. She or he may take forever to decide what to order, place countless special conditions on the order (dressing on the side, no butter or oil, hold the croutons), and then spend the mealtime picking at the food and being silenced by anxiety and fear. The entire social aspect of sharing a meal becomes consumed by the controlling nature of the eating disorder.

Worse things can happen, too. I recall a patient who was mortified by an experience she had when she and her husband went out to dinner with another couple and had decided in advance that they would split the bill to avoid any haggling.

Rose was recovering from bulimia and thought she was at a point where she could handle a meal in a restaurant, if she was able to access the menu ahead of time online and do some careful planning. She checked out the menu in advance and that evening proceeded to order what she thought was a safe meal. What she hadn't factored into the equation was how a glass of wine with dinner would affect her appetite and her feelings about what she had eaten. She excused herself after dinner and went to the ladies' room absolutely paralyzed by the fear of what she had consumed. Unbeknownst to Rose, her friend had followed her into the restroom and overheard Rose when she could no longer combat the urge to purge. She stayed behind in the stall, absolutely mortified, until her friend went back to the table. When Rose returned, her husband squeezed her hand in attempt to comfort her, guessing what had happened. But clearly her friend had told her own husband what had happened because when it came time to split the bill, he said, "There's no way I'm gonna split this bill. Rose just barfed up everything she ate . . . that's a waste of my money." The need for serious sensitivity training aside, this type of interaction can and does happen when acquaintances simply have no clue what eating disorders are all about.

Going out to dinner with people who don't have eating disorders can also be highly triggering for people who have active disorders or who are in recovery. Typical mealtime chatter is often like a play-by-play of tastes, textures, and presentations. If you have bulimia or BED, sitting at a table with a group of people who are savoring, "yumming," discussing every detail of the food, and pushing you to taste it is the same type of experience that a barely abstinent ex-smoker has if someone takes a deep drag of a cigarette and exclaims how great it feels to inhale deeply and fill his lungs with menthol, or if an alcoholic goes to a bar and everyone is describing how good that first drink feels going down. Or, if you have anorexia, it's like having a height phobia, being in a helicopter with no doors, and having the pilot tilt the machine to make you look down and dangle your feet.

It's not just the food or the discussion about the food that can be triggering, however. People have no idea how their normal chatter about weight and appetite can ignite a tailspin in someone with an eating disorder. Here are some seemingly innocuous comments that could be highly triggering: "I haven't eaten all day to make room for this," "I couldn't eat another bite if I tried," "Is that all you're going to eat?" "This dessert is so worth the three hours on the treadmill." Let's break these "innocent" comments down and hear what the person with an eating disorder actually hears.

First, "I haven't eaten all day to make room for this." This comment could trigger someone in recovery from anorexia nervosa to become competitive about how much she is eating. She always wants to be the one who eats least, so this could make her feel as if she hadn't punished herself enough by restricting before going out to dinner. Second, "I couldn't eat another bite if I tried." A person with BED might rebel internally and say, "Ha! You have no idea what someone is capable of eating," which could set off a binge as soon as he got home. Finally, "This dessert is so worth the three hours on the treadmill" is enough to inspire calorie math in someone with any eating disorder and be the impetus for a bout of overexercising or caloric restriction as payback for eating dessert.

In no way am I saying that we have to tiptoe around someone with an eating disorder. In fact, a very important part of recovery is learning how to navigate the complicated waters of normal conversation and comments about eating and appearance. The point is that an eating disorder can disrupt the very threads from which relationships are woven. Hardly a social occasion takes place that doesn't involve food or alcohol, and the tension surrounding food and alcohol can cause people with eating disorders to detach from critically important aspects of their lives.

Impact on Work

A fundamental difference between adult and adolescent eating disorders is the impact on work. A number of very enlightening studies have revealed the extent to which eating disorders influence daily functioning and productivity. Many metrics have been developed to describe this effect, and concepts such as "disability days" are used by the National Comorbidity Study in the United States to determine the extent to which symptoms or clusters of symptoms affect everyday functioning.[24]

Australian studies have clarified just how disabling eating disorders are in adults. One study explored the impact of self-induced vomiting, laxatives, diuretics, restriction, binge eating, and excessive exercise on daily functioning and found that, of these symptoms, self-induced vomiting was associated with the greatest impairment and distress. In fact, nearly half of the cases surveyed were "severely" disabled according to their metric, which is comparable to the impact of depression and anxiety.[25] This is particularly noteworthy given that depression has the highest ranking globally of all health conditions for years lost due to disability.[26]

In another study, those who reported regular eating disorder behaviors (including binge eating, purging, and fasting) had higher levels of functional impairment and "days out of role" than those who did not. That means, they were unable to complete work, school, or household responsibilities because of problems with their physical or emotional health. Of interest, individuals who reported greater concerns about their shape and weight also reported greater impairment.[27]

While it's not clear exactly how eating disorders impair work functioning, our observations in the clinic provide some clues. Dieting and food restriction can affect concentration through the effects of starvation. People with anorexia nervosa perform more poorly on tests of simple reaction time and recalling events and objects,[28] indicating impaired concentration. Typically, these skills return after recovery,[29] but they can seriously interfere with performance during active illness. In addition, all eating disorders are characterized by preoccupying and often obsessional thoughts, whether about body shape and size or about eating and food. People with anorexia and bulimia report significantly more negative thoughts about themselves and their bodies when looking in a mirror, weighing themselves, and indulging in a chocolate treat than those without eating disorders.[30] The types of thoughts include fears about "getting fatter and fatter" and having "no self-control."

Somewhat paradoxically, despite their unwillingness to eat, or perhaps because of this unwillingness, individuals with anorexia nervosa are constantly thinking about food. The roots of this could lie in some basic evolutionary advantage. Keeping food in the front of your mind during times of famine could serve to enhance your vigilance for food sources and motivate searching for sustenance. The stereotypes of individuals with anorexia nervosa are true: The majority do often collect recipes, watch cooking shows on TV, and enjoy cooking for others, but they just don't eat themselves. For both similar and different reasons, individuals with bulimia nervosa and BED also spend a lot of time thinking about food. This preoccupation can directly interfere with the amount of brain space they have available for work- or school-related thoughts and directly impair performance.

Beyond the effect of actually binge eating and purging on daily functioning, just the urge to engage in these behaviors can affect concentration and performance. Someone with bulimia or BED might become completely overwhelmed by an urge to binge. Even with other tasks piling up, the brain can be pulled back into the vortex that is compelling them to binge or purge. These thoughts can be all-consuming and leave few mental reserves for work-related activities. Even if the person yields to these urges and binges or purges on the job, afterward, guilt or shame can rush in to occupy that brain space, further detracting from the ability to concentrate on the task at hand.

Elena, for example, recalled a day when work-related stress was particularly high as her company prepared for an audit. The vending machine on the first floor kept beckoning her with thoughts of chocolate . . . and lots of it, drowning out her audit-related tasks. She was staring at pieces of paper, trying to organize materials, but finding her thoughts completely fixated on chocolate. Elena finally gave up, left her office, went down to the vending machine, and quickly inhaled not one but six chocolate bars. She returned to her office hoping that, with the chocolate obsession out of her system, she might be able to finally get her work done. Yet, as she set out to organize the paperwork, all Elena could do was think about how disgusting she was for having lost control.

Body image thoughts can also interfere with concentration. Although most women have frequent thoughts related to body dissatisfaction throughout the day, this is magnified in women with eating disorders. The same is true in men, although the discrepancy is particularly striking between healthy men, who are much less likely to be preoccupied with their bodies than women, and men with eating disorders. These negative body thoughts don't just occur during trips to the ladies' or men's room when you catch a glimpse of yourself in the mirror; these are constant nagging thoughts about body dissatisfaction, which can be triggered by comparison with other people, by glancing down at various body parts, by physical sensations after eating, or by just about any thought or memory. The important point is that all these thoughts are filling the brains of individuals with eating disorders and impairing their ability to concentrate, which has obvious implications for productivity and effectiveness on the job.

Carlos watched several less qualified colleagues get promoted and receive plum assignments while he was perpetually stuck with low-impact tasks. In his heart of hearts, he knew that it was because he could not contain his thoughts about eating during the workday. In addition, the number of sick days he had taken after episodes of binging had flagged him as a "problem employee." This resulted in Carlos's immediate supervisor working with him on a remediation plan to decrease absenteeism and improve job performance. Although he was mortified at being singled out and labeled in this way, he was too ashamed to seek treatment for his eating disorder for fear that his physician would not understand that men suffer from eating disorders, too.

Eating disorders, or any disordered eating behavior, can

impair other functions that are critical to job performance. Many people with eating disorders are less effective at tolerating stress, which can make typical workplace challenges overwhelming to individuals whose only, or primary, method of dealing with stress is food, starvation, or exercise—none of which is helpful in the middle of the workday. Binge eating at your desk or skipping lunch are clearly ineffective at relieving stress, and it's not always possible to get to hot yoga. This inability to be effective in the face of stress can lead to job stagnation and to missed opportunities, creating a cycle of dissatisfaction and more, rather than less, stress.

We can also assess the impact of disordered eating on other brain-controlled functions. Using a simple tapping test that tallies how quickly individuals can punch the numbers one and two on a keyboard two hundred times, researchers found that people with anorexia nervosa were slower than healthy individuals.[31] Even this simple test suggests that in our keyboard-dependent society, anorexia can have direct effects on performance. It's not just these simple motor skills that are impaired; higher brain functions are also affected. Using a test called the Gambling Task, researchers explored how well individuals can balance immediate rewards against long-term negative consequences, which is a type of decision making that occurs regularly, including in the workplace. Women with anorexia nervosa were poorer in decision making than healthy women, and their poor performance was not fully explained by how ill they were at the time of testing. What's more, these cognitive deficits do not necessarily return to normal with treatment.[32] The researchers involved with this work believe that poor decision making in unrelated tasks mirrors the poor decision making of people with anorexia when it comes to food. When hungry, they actively choose to avoid eating in order to reduce their anxiety about eating and weight gain (i.e., immediate reward) while failing to balance the long-term negative consequences of their decision, such as declining physical health and potential death. Michael Strober, Ph.D., and Craig Johnson, Ph.D., two of the forefathers of the eating disorders field, explain, "We do our best to warn patients that they are feeling the pull of misguided ideas, but they are tone deaf to the standard logic applied to health."[33] I would change that statement to say that patients may very well understand the logic applied to health, but they just don't think that logic applies to them.

The Financial Toll of Midlife Eating Disorders

Eating disorders are expensive both to have and to treat. The disorders themselves exact a financial toll via binge foods, laxatives, supplements, and gym memberships (see the box on page 62) while, on the treatment end, the cost of specialized inpatient care or residential treatment programs ranges from fifteen hundred dollars to more than two thousand dollars per day, with duration of stay varying from weeks to months.[34] Even partial hospitalization programs advertise rates from five hundred to fifteen hundred dollars per day. Outpatient treatment often combines treatment from several health care providers and can include primary care and psychiatrist appointments, psychotherapy, and dietary counseling, which may not all be covered by health insurance. Inadequate insurance coverage and high copays can place an inordinate burden on families of adults with midlife eating disorders. When treatment is available only at facilities far from home, the travel costs for the patient and family members further add to the accumulating costs of the eating disorder.

A report prepared in 2012 by the UK advocacy group Beating Eating Disorders (beat) in conjunction with the London-based charity Pro Bono Economics, carefully estimated the economic impact of eating disorders by considering both direct health care costs as well as the impact on gross domestic product via reduced productivity, earnings, and other intangibles.

The report estimated the following costs related to eating disorders.

* More than £80 million ($125 million) as the value of health care treatment costs;
* More than £230 million ($360 million) as the present value of reduced gross domestic product (GDP);
* More than £950 million ($1.49 billion) as the value of reduced length of life and health

This makes a total of over £1.25 billion ($1.96 billion) in costs for England per year—and this total is based on conservative estimates.[35]

In describing the financial impact of his wife's eating disorder, Rob lamented, "We had always planned on getting the kids through college, taking a nice cruise in the Mediterranean to celebrate that milestone, and then retiring to a warmer climate. But after three inpatient stays, two residential treatments, and all of the outpatient therapy, we have eaten through our financial reserves, exhausted our retirement funds, and taken out a second mortgage on our home. Even if she lives, we'll never take that cruise, and we'll never be able to afford to retire."

Stories like these are all too familiar as insurance companies balk at covering the cost of the long-term intervention required for successful treatment of some eating disorders. Unfortunately, when an insurance company drops the ball on coverage, active lobbying by patients or partners is required. As detailed in an investigative piece in the *New York Times*, the burden is often on the patient or partner to fight the initial denial of coverage.[36] The first stop is a case manager, who may or may not be able to assist. The second stop is a member of the employer's human resources department, who may be able to advocate on behalf of the patient. If there's still no movement, patients and families may need to contact their state's insurance commissioner or their congressional representative. This may seem overwhelming during times of suffering or crisis, but it's better to put forth the effort to obtain adequate coverage for treatment than to be financially devastated and have to relinquish dreams, like Rob and his family. There is no question that the squeaky wheel gets the attention in this situation.

ANNUALIZED COSTS OF BINGE EATING AND PURGING

Scott Crow, M.D., and colleagues from the University of Minnesota were interested in how much bulimia nervosa actually costs in terms of annual expenditure for binge foods and purgatives such as laxatives, diuretics, and diet pills.[37] To determine this, they asked ten women with bulimia to complete very detailed records for several days: to write down everything they ate, when they binged and purged, and how many laxatives, diuretics, or diet pills they took. On average, these women reported binge eating 4.9 times per week and purging 3.6 times per week. The researchers then separated the cost of binge and non-binge foods and found that, in an average week, these women spent between $7 and $67 on binge foods. Likewise, they spent between $0 and $28 on purgatives and diet pills. Combining expenditures and annualizing the information, these women spent between $368 and $4,954 dollars per year sustaining their bulimia. The top of that range is about the equivalent of a three-pack-a-day cigarette habit at $6 per pack. This research suggests that a prolonged case of bulimia with an average duration of illness of 12.9 years, and taking into account only the costs of binge foods and purgatives, can add up to nearly $64,000! That amount of cash can be an enormous drain on personal and family resources and is often not accounted for when considering the financial toll of eating disorders.

AWARENESS AND ACTION

We all have a voice, yet we rarely speak out against things we see or experience that infuriate us. Whether corporations will listen to anything but profit margins depends on the circumstances, but some media watchdog groups have had impressive success in getting corporations to reverse bad marketing strategies. It is harder to do this as a lone voice, but you can help by feeding your observations to groups that do have the power and influence to create change. The National Eating Disorders Association (NEDA) has a Media Watchdog group that anyone can join. It has a Facebook page on which group members can point out ads that are offensive or detrimental to people with eating disorders (http://www.facebook.com/groups/41474787925). According to NEDA, Media Watchdogs are volunteers who advocate for responsible, healthy messaging in various forms of media, commending or critiquing advertisements or programs that positively or negatively impact body image and self-concept. Watchdogs pay attention to TV, radio, newspaper, magazine, and Internet ads or programs, send notices of those worthy of praise or protest to the NEDA office, and alert other Watchdogs of potential actions through the Media Watchdogs Facebook Group.[38] Since its launch in 1997, more than half of the protested advertisements targeted by NEDA's Media Watchdog program have been pulled, including a recent commercial for Yoplait Light yogurt that highlighted a woman experiencing disordered thoughts while deciding whether to eat a piece of cheesecake as a reward for having been "good," and bargaining to balance out the cheesecake by eating it with celery sticks or by consuming it while jogging in place.[39]

To start using your voice, be aware of the advertisements around you and, if you find a praise- or protest-worthy one, submit it to the NEDA Media Watchdog office. Only by joining our voices can we create change.

CHAPTER 4

The Face of Eating Disorders in Men

Kristen recounted a horrifying story from her days in graduate school. One of her psych nursing professors, a man, was very skinny. He was a very engaging professor, a conscientious grader, and passionate about psych nursing, but she recalled the class gossip mill constantly debating whether he had cancer or AIDS, or whether he was just one of those naturally thin people who could eat anything he wanted. Anorexia nervosa crossed their minds, but they were quick to rule it out because he was a guy in his thirties. They often saw him running around campus, so marathoner was added to the list of possible explanations for his physique. One Monday morning, he didn't show up for class. After about fifteen minutes of waiting, just as they were all about to leave, the dean entered the classroom and informed them that their professor had died over the weekend from cardiac arrest secondary to anorexia nervosa. Kristen was horrified that they had all basically watched him waste away before their very eyes, and that it had happened in a nursing school, where he had been teaching psychiatric nursing courses, and no one had seemed to catch on—just because he was a man.

Men of all ages, all shapes and sizes, all sexual orientations, and all races and ethnicities develop eating disorders. They, perhaps even more than their female counterparts, face enormous stigmatization that can inhibit them from seeking treatment and receiving adequate care. Further complicating our understanding of eating disorders in men is the fact that eating disorders have been defined around women. This is the reverse of what we typically see in medicine, where the majority of testing and recommendations are based on clinical trials of adult men. At the most fundamental level, even our basic definitions of eating disorders are crafted around their presentations in women.

Getting a handle on just how common eating disorders are in men is a challenge, and the data are conflicting. Surveying more than eighteen hundred men in the northwestern United States, Dr. Ruth Striegel and her colleagues found fairly high rates of disordered eating in those between the ages of eighteen and thirty-five.[1] Men reported overeating (26 percent), losing control while eating (20 percent), and binge eating at least once per week (8 percent). In order to avoid weight gain after binge eating, they also engaged in a variety of compensatory behaviors, including purging (1.5 percent), fasting for 24 or more hours (4 percent), taking more than twice the recommended dose of laxatives (3 percent), and exercising for more than one hour (5.6 percent).

Men report somewhat less dissatisfaction with their bodies and less drive for thinness than women, which may be due to their greater concern with leanness and muscularity than weight loss per se. There are some striking inconsistencies that we do not yet understand. A study of Puerto Rican college students revealed higher rates of binge eating and compensatory behaviors (laxative use, vomiting, and diuretic use) in men than in women.[2]

The best epidemiologic data that we have in the United States surveyed more than nine thousand households and revealed a lifetime prevalence in men of 0.3 percent for anorexia nervosa, 0.5 percent for bulimia nervosa, and 2 percent for BED.[3] Not surprisingly, the majority of men with eating disorders suffered from at least one other psychological disorder, including mood, anxiety, impulse-control, and/or substance use disorders.

Turning these percentages into real numbers reveals that approximately 3.2 million men over the age of eighteen have suffered from anorexia, bulimia, or BED. Adding in other estimates we have from EDNOS and purging disorder brings the total up to around 3.8 million men in the United States. Clearly, we need to pay far more attention to eating disorders in boys and men.

The 2007 Adult Psychiatric Morbidity Survey (APMS) conducted in the United Kingdom also administered the SCOFF screening questionnaire to men and identified the following percentages of men who screened positive for eating disorders: age 16 to 24 (1.7 percent); 25 to 34 (0.7 percent); 35 to 44 (0.3 percent); 45 to 54 (0.8 percent); 55 to 64 (0.1 percent); and 65 to 74 (0.3 percent). Overall 0.6 percent of men screened positive for eating disorders by this definition, translating roughly into 125,000 men in the United Kingdom.[4]

Two Australian surveys conducted ten years apart also show increases in symptoms of eating disorders in men. The 1995 study reported the following prevalences in men in the state of South Australia: 3.1 percent for binge eating, 0 percent for purging, and 0.6 percent for strict dieting or fasting. Ten years later, as in the parallel study on women, each of these estimates more than doubled, reaching 7.8 percent binge eating, 1 percent purging, and 3.9 percent strict dieting or fasting.[5]

Clinical Presentation in Men
To address the clinical presentation in men, we have to ask two questions: What's the same? And what's different? On the side of similarities, it is not uncommon for anorexia nervosa, bulimia nervosa, purging disorder, and BED to look functionally similar in men and women. The symptoms, comorbid conditions, course, and outcome can and do follow the same pattern.

In terms of differences, the nature of body dissatisfaction can drive men and women in opposite directions, resulting in quite different symptoms. We observed striking differences in the type and function of compensatory behaviors across genders. The frequency of "prototypical" behaviors (e.g., self-induced vomiting, laxative abuse) was lower in men, but the frequency of non-purging behaviors (e.g., excessive exercise, supplement use) was higher in men. Men and women may compensate in different ways.[6] As we have discussed, women compensate primarily to achieve weight reduction. Although some men compensate for weight reduction, others may focus on decreasing body fat, and others actually on gaining weight or increasing muscle mass. Unfortunately, DSM-IV and DSM-5 fail to capture the variety of compensatory behaviors we can see in men with eating disorders. Moreover, DSM-IV defines the purpose of compensatory behaviors as being "to prevent weight gain." This failure to acknowledge why some men engage in behaviors with an altogether different goal may perpetuate the underdetection and underrecognition of eating disorders in men.

If we look at the psychosocial roots of body dissatisfaction, these gender differences are consistent with Western body image stereotypes. Since the 1950s, cultural norms have driven women toward dieting and weight loss to meet the culturally determined thin ideal. For men, cultural pressures are in the opposite direction, namely toward increased body mass, particularly muscle mass. While the Barbie doll's proportions were distorting to unattainable dimensions, the G.I. Joe doll attained a degree of muscularity that would simply encumber a living being. Compounding the challenge to men, although muscle mass ideals are increasing, waist size ideals are not. So just like Barbie, G.I. Joe would basically snap in the middle if his minuscule waist had to carry around all of that upper-body bulk.

There is a second type of body ideal that can lure men

down dangerous weight control paths. In contrast to the muscle-laden jock body is the equally alluring heroin-chic, glam-rock, hipster-thin, rehab-bound, androgynous-looking male-model physique, which rivals the female runway model in its lack of muscularity. The fashion industry has both followed and led this trend, with Japanese designers on the forefront portraying men as slender, vulnerable, and in need of protection. Describing this trend in the *New York Times*, Kaori Shoji claims that men are "espousing an emaciated, tragic sexiness" and giving off the vibe that they want to be "fed and/or devoured by women."[7] This tubercular ideal, quite opposite from the beefed-up muscular ideal, can lure men into very similar extreme weight control approaches as women. Especially in those men who are genetically at greater risk, striving for this emaciated ideal can unhinge a cascade of disordered eating and dieting behaviors that result in anorexia nervosa.

Because this is an ideal, and because of the widespread misconception that there are men out there who "can eat whatever they want and not gain weight," men with anorexia nervosa often go unnoticed. As in the case of the nursing professor cited at the beginning of this chapter, friends, family, and physicians will come up with scores of explanations for weight loss before they even consider anorexia nervosa as a possibility in men. The data disagree. We are doing a huge disservice to the sufferers, their partners, and their families by failing to detect and treat anorexia nervosa in boys and men.

In the best of all possible diagnostic worlds, our descriptions of eating disorders would explain body dissatisfaction and compensatory behaviors in a manner that is congruent with these culturally driven ideals and allow for gender differences. This broader diagnostic view would not only include the drive for thinness but also would make room for the drive for leanness or the drive for muscularity—thus capturing the true range of body dissatisfaction seen across the sexes.

MY EATING DISORDER WAS INVISIBLE

Mark Warren, M.D., M.P.H., FAED, is the chief medical officer and chief operating officer of the Cleveland Center for Eating Disorders. He can attest to the invisibility of eating disorders in many men. He recalls, "What stands out for me most in my experience of my eating disorder was how completely invisible the disorder was. I didn't know I was ill, no one else ever knew I was ill, not a single comment was ever directed to me about eating disorders. This was despite a significant weight loss, low BMI, an ER visit, bradycardia (slow heart rate), obsessive exercise, and bizarre restrictive eating patterns. To be a man with a girl's disease put me miles off the radar. As I talk to others who have had eating disorders in their history, I feel like I had an absolute textbook case of anorexia nervosa and was fortunate to have a variation of the illness that was treatable by refeeding (by my wife), behavioral change, therapy, and a supportive community. I never tried to get formal treatment for the disorder, but that was because I was blind to it. I did carry a lot of shame about who I was, not being perfect, and of course, about my body. I carried some shame about having a disease associated with women, but that was only after the fact. While the illness was on me, I didn't even know I had it. If we are going to get more men to get into treatment for their eating disorders, then the first step is to make sure that the illness is seen by families and professionals. With good treatment there is good reason to have hope for recovery."

Binge Eating in Men
Anorexia nervosa is not the only eating disorder that we know precious little about in men. In fact, if you look at clinical trials for all of the eating disorders, men are completely underrepresented. In the majority of treatment studies—in fact in studies

of eating disorders, period—you will often see a disclaimer such as, "Due to the small number of men identified, they were excluded from the analysis." Wondering why men were typically underrepresented in clinical trials and treatment settings for eating disorders, psychologist Ruth Striegel, Ph.D., and her team explored whether binge eating in men was simply associated with less impairment, thereby making men less likely to seek treatment: in other words, maybe they binged but just didn't care. This was far from the case. In studying more than forty-five thousand individuals, they found that binge eating in both men and women was associated with higher BMI, greater depression and stress, lower work productivity, and daily health-related nonwork impairment. Smaller differences also emerged around sleep problems, hypertension, dyslipidemia (high cholesterol or fat in the blood), and Type 2 diabetes, with individuals who binge ate indicating more impairment on all of these dimensions. Men and women who reported binge eating were also more likely to miss work due to illness. Thus, binge eating is as concerning in men as it is in women, but lack of awareness and failure to seek treatment are the most likely culprits for their underrepresentation in the clinic.[8]

Risk Factors for Eating Disorders in Men
Genetic Factors. Although the majority of genetic studies of eating disorders have been conducted in women, we have no reason to believe that genetic factors play any less of a role in men. One report revealed that female relatives of males with anorexia nervosa are more than twenty times as likely to have anorexia nervosa themselves than relatives of males without anorexia nervosa.[9] This strong family clustering could mean that genetic factors play a substantial role in males. We have also shown that binge eating is equally as heritable in men as in women and some of the same genetic factors seem to be at play.[10] Although the data are scarce, it is imperative that we attend to the role of genes in all eating disorders in men.

Bullying and Teasing. Whereas many of the purported risk factors for eating disorders in men are similar to those for women, a few stand out as especially poignant for men. Ted Weltzin, M.D., medical director of the Eating Disorder Services Center at Wisconsin's Rogers Memorial Hospital—the only residential program in the United States with a specific treatment program for men—emphasizes the role of teasing and bullying at the root of eating disorders in many men. They recall taunts about weight and lack of strength, being called wimps or nerds or any number of other names that young boys can call each other. In Dr. Weltzin's practice, these are common triggers for male eating disorders and underscore just how destructive they can be. Dr. Weltzin is also careful to say that teasing and bullying are not specific causes of eating disorders, but rather are nonspecific risk factors that can lead to a range of problems, including depression, anxiety, and alcohol and drug abuse.

Dr. Weltzin carries his observations one step farther, explaining that invalidating responses by parents or teachers to reports of bullying can also intensify the impact that this harassment has on the development of eating disorders. When parents respond with comments like "Oh, just don't let it get to you," or "Man up and deal with it," they fail to empathize with how traumatizing and isolating bullying can be. Dr. Weltzin shares that, in their recovery journeys, many men who were teased or bullied are very determined "to never go back there," to that horrible trap of being harassed about weight or sexuality, or whatever the target was. Bullying leaves lifelong scars that these men try to heal, or at least conceal, with their eating disordered behaviors.

Men relate how weight-based victimization can cut to the core of men's ability to deal with their moods and can compromise their core sense of identity. Men with eating disorders may feel weak or lazy if they don't lose as much weight as they want, guilty about not living up to expectations, and angry about feeling misunderstood. Dr. Weltzin explains that men who come into treatment often initially address eating disorder behaviors, followed by depression, social avoidance, and low self-esteem, and then finally develop a healthy sense of self-esteem as it relates to their unique individual talents and interests.

Sports with a Weight Focus. Another high-risk environment for eating disorders in men is the sports arena, where women aren't the only victims of the "thin to win" mentality. Participants in several male sports run a high risk for disordered eating. "The lighter you are, the farther you fly," is the motto of male ski jumpers.[11] If you watch winter sports, you'll remember back in the 1980s when the V-technique became popular. Before that, men jumped with their ski tips close together and parallel. With the advent of the V-technique, where the tips are spread in front to create a V shape, the jumper's weight became a critical component to the aerodynamics of jumping: losing a single kilogram (2.2 pounds) can translate into an additional 6.5 to 13 feet in jumping distance, leading male ski jumpers to extreme weight loss in order to achieve a competitive advantage.[12] The International Ski Federation enacted rules in 2004 that tied maximum ski length, another crucial variable, to the jumper's BMI.[13] The rules now go so far as to allow a maximum ski length of 145 percent of height only for male jumpers with a BMI of 21 or above. Any male jumper whose BMI is under 21 is actually penalized 0.5 percent in maximum ski length per 0.125 BMI units below the threshold.

Success in competitive horse racing has long been tied to jockeys staying light enough to comply with maximum weights set by individual racetracks, which are based on the type of race and the horse's age, sex, and past performances, and are designed to reduce stress and potential injury in the horse.[14] Although the weight limit is one hundred twenty-six pounds for the Kentucky Derby, it may be ten or even fifteen pounds less for other races. Not surprisingly, jockeys often resort to extreme weight-loss techniques to comply with these limits, including vomiting and endless hours in the sauna. Locker rooms at racetracks even provide "heave bowls" and "hot boxes" to support these dangerous practices, which put jockeys at higher risk for esophagitis, osteoporosis, heart problems, dental issues, electrolyte disturbances, drug addiction, and even death. Beginning in 2005, racetracks in several states, including California, Florida, Kentucky, New Jersey, and New York, raised minimum weights to one hundred fifteen to one hundred sixteen pounds, and at the North American Racing Academy in Lexington, Kentucky, there is a mandatory nutrition course to teach jockeys about healthy dietary habits. In 2009, the National Institute for Occupational Safety and Health issued a game-changing report regarding workplace safety for jockeys in response to a congressional inquiry that provides recommendations for reducing the number of injuries and adverse health effects for workers in the horse-racing industry.[15]

One look at all of the cyclists clustered in the peloton of any cycling race will tell you that there are many male cyclists who are below a healthy body weight. Cycling places tremendous emphasis on attaining a lean body and low weight, as a high power-to-weight ratio is linked to racing success.[16] A recent study showed that male cyclists scored significantly higher on measures of disordered eating, dieting, bulimia, and food preoccupation than controls. Eating disorders were also more common, and a dietary questionnaire revealed that few of the cyclists were meeting the caloric needs necessary for their intense training regimens. Together, these trends may put cyclists at risk for a range of negative health outcomes, including osteoporosis, vitamin deficiencies, hormone and electrolyte imbalances, stress fractures, and even death.

The National Eating Disorders Association (NEDA) estimates that 33 percent of male athletes in "aesthetic sports" (e.g., bodybuilding, gymnastics, diving) and "weight-class sports" (e.g., wrestling, light-weight rowing, horse racing) suffer from eating disorders, but the psychological and physical stresses placed on competitive athletes in any sport can increase their risk for disordered eating.[17] Wrestlers, in particular, are known for resorting to a variety of tactics to "make weight" before matches, including calorie and fluid restriction, binging and purging, laxative and diuretic abuse, and excessive exercise.[18] This is often in attempt to compete in the lowest possible weight class for their size, giving them a supposed strength advantage. Post-match celebrations can devolve into group binges, and the off-season is often marked with dramatic weight regain.

Men's "Health" Magazines and Advertising. I have vivid memories of reading *Reader's Digest* as a young girl when the series "I am Joe's [insert body part]" appeared. I remember reading about Joe's lung and Joe's heart, and then eventually some articles about Jane appeared as well. Back in the day, this was how health information was disseminated to the general public. Recently I picked up some of today's men's health and fitness magazines to see what men were being exposed to and whether the Big Industries were trying to make men feel as bad about themselves as women are. What a shocker! I learned that, to be attractive to the opposite sex as a man, you have to be completely hairless (except for a meticulously cultivated and oddly shaped five o'clock shadow) or expertly "manscaped," have somewhere between six- and twelve-pack abs, have a V-shaped torso, smell good even when you sweat, be a total sex machine, never get tired, drive a hot car, work hard in the gym to drop pounds and build lean muscle, go from weakling to crusher, love meat but eat more vegetarian, and, by all means, wear a very big and very expensive watch. That is today's definition of what a man "should" be.

If I were a guy, I would feel as inadequate reading these rags as women do when they read their own magazines. I would wonder about these other men who have somehow been born with miraculously perfect hair distributions and perfectly formed, appropriately sized nipples. I would feel as if I "should" drop pounds, build sculpted muscles, get ripped abs, and become an ironman, a warrior, a prime man. These magazines, just like those for women, are setting impossible standards for men to strive for and are marketing expensive placebos, gadgets, and equipment to achieve them, which are purported not only to boost a man's body esteem but also his self-esteem. By targeting younger and younger men and boys, industries are implanting the same sort of dissatisfaction mind worms in men's heads as they do in women's, no doubt fueling all kinds of inappropriate weight-loss and muscle-gaining behaviors. There is no question that Photoshop is as widely applied in men's magazines as in women's—but in the other direction. Instead of just making waists and thighs smaller, advertisers make waists smaller and thighs and biceps bigger. Moreover, the industry is equally guilty of trying to convince older gentlemen that they needn't exhibit any visible signs of aging—that youth is just around the corner. A magic cocktail of Viagra and human growth hormone could keep them as fit and strong as a champion, a warrior, and an alpha male, well into their seventies and eighties. We need to recognize that these messages are just as damaging and infectious as those that have haunted women for decades.

Physical Effects of Eating Disorders on Men
In addition to the physical complications outlined in the table starting on page 44 in Chapter 3, there are some additional health concerns specific to men with eating disorders. In the general population, osteoporosis (thinning bones) is more common in women. This is largely due to several factors, namely that men lay down greater skeletal bone mass during youth, have a larger bone size, do not go through menopause, and live somewhat shorter lives than women. Testosterone, the primary

male sex hormone, plays a key role in the maintenance of bone mass, and low testosterone can be associated with osteoporosis in men. Testosterone levels are decreased in men with both anorexia and bulimia nervosa, with the lowest levels seen in men with the restricting subtype of anorexia nervosa.[19] Low testosterone is also associated with decreased sex drive and impaired sexual performance.

Men with anorexia nervosa may actually be at higher risk of developing osteoporosis than their female counterparts, with 78 percent of men with restricting anorexia nervosa, 75 percent of men with anorexia nervosa of the binge/purge subtype, 50 percent of men with bulimia nervosa, and 25 percent of men with EDNOS being afflicted. The bone loss in these men was actually more severe than in women with anorexia. This study also raised significant concerns about prolonged bone loss in boys and men, as they might be at increased risk for fractures, even after recovery.[20]

Although data on mortality due to eating disorders in men are limited, one study suggested that deaths from anorexia nervosa are more likely to occur within the first two years of presentation, whereas deaths in women with anorexia nervosa continued over time.[21] Men actually report more adverse health consequences from BED than do women.[22]

Emotional Avoidance

One of the traps for many men is how they process or fail to process their emotions. Thomas Joiner, Ph.D., the Bright-Burton Professor of Psychology at Florida State University, has dealt extensively with how things can go wrong with men. In his book *Lonely at the Top: The High Cost of Men's Success*,[23] he describes how men can let relationships take a backseat to their professional ambitions, then wake up and find themselves bereft of true connections with others and ways to deal with their emotions. This fundamental loneliness can lead to affairs, depression, alcohol, self-destructive behaviors, suicide, and, of course, eating disorders. Dr. Joiner states that "ignoring relationships in favor of things and outcomes . . . facilitates the taking for granted of relationships that characterizes men more than women . . . [this] is a main source for male loneliness and all the woe that comes with it."

Our society has coerced men and boys into believing that it is not acceptable to express a whole palette of emotions typically associated with being female. It's acceptable for them to express anger, but exposing emotions such as sadness, anxiety, nervousness, and tenderness puts them straight into the firing line of being criticized for not being sufficiently masculine.

Dr. Ted Weltzin folds this observation directly into his clinical experience and cites evidence that one of the primary functions of eating disorders in men is emotional avoidance. The yellow crime-scene tape around emotions drives men to avoid their natural emotional responses and, instead, turn to food—whether that be avoidance of food and seeking control via restriction, or avoiding emotions by binge eating. We do our sons no favors when we tell them "not to feel" certain emotions, which paves the way to avoidance of critical aspects of the human experience that can transform into eating disorders or into other problems such as drug or alcohol abuse.

In treating bulimia nervosa effectively, one core tenet is to identify the thoughts and feelings that can trigger binge eating or purging. Although it is often challenging for patients of both sexes to separate thoughts and feelings, and to identify specific feelings that may act as triggers, men, at least in the initial phases of treatment, can have a particularly difficult time even acknowledging that feelings might be triggers. When asked about feelings that could trigger a binge, Peter, age thirty-eight, said, "There aren't any feelings, it's just habit." After a few months of therapy, he reflected back on his early self-monitoring and said, "I really was a bulimic automaton, or at least I convinced myself that I was. I had stuffed all of the feelings that I now recognize right down my throat and convinced myself it was just a bad habit that I had to get over. Now I know there is more work—more emotional work—to do in order to break this cycle." He went on to say, "Remember how hesitant I was to be in a group with women? Well, now I am kind of glad I was; they wouldn't let me get away with deluding myself into thinking my emotions weren't involved."

On the Periphery of Eating Disorders
In addition to the classic eating disorders, there are a variety of related disturbing behaviors and syndromes that occur in men, such as preoccupation with shape and weight, purging, and the use of supplements to alter appearance. Tom Hildebrandt, Psy.D. of Mount Sinai Medical Center in New York City, has contributed enormously to our understanding of the breadth and nature of these problems in men. He clarifies that eating disorders in men can often be obscured behind the pursuit of athletic achievement, health, and/or perfect appearance. Unlike the pervasive "thin ideal" for women, the physical appearance goals in men may differ, ranging from the same classic desire for thinness to reverse goals of bodybuilding or a drive for the low-body-fat, intense muscularity of an underwear model. Other men may become fixated on or obsessed with reaching fitness goals without focusing much on their actual weight.

Dr. Hildebrandt regularly sees deliberate severe caloric restriction, excessive exercise or training, purposeful overeating (often done under rigid dietary control—for example, eating five thousand calories in a day, but 80 percent from protein with carbs only right before a workout), purging, anabolic-androgenic steroid abuse, and serial supplement use in order to achieve a desired physical or fitness goal.

Supplements. All of these unhealthy behaviors may interact and converge into more extreme shape- and weight-controlling behaviors such as the use of supplements and illegal substances to change appearance. Dr. Hildebrandt warns that the more of these symptoms that are present (over-exercise, perfectionism, shape and weight concerns), the greater likelihood that an individual also uses fitness supplements (e.g., β-hydroxy β-methylbutyric acid (HMB), amino acids, creatine, etc.) and anabolic-androgenic steroids (AASs). Supplements and AASs can be confused by the novice because the legally available fitness supplements are often marketed as if they were the more potent and illegal AASs. Frighteningly, in the absence of regulation by the Food and Drug Administration, up to 10 percent of these supplements are contaminated with illegal substances, but they are seen as "safe" by the user because they are legal.

Steroid Use. AASs are synthetic hormones derived from natural sex hormones that fall under the umbrella of appearance- and performance-enhancing drugs (APEDs), which also include nonsteroidal anabolics (human growth hormone or HGH, insulin), ancillary drugs (human chorionic gonadotropin or HCG, Viagra), nutritional supplements (creatine, protein powder), and stimulants, weight-loss drugs, or endurance drugs (ephedrine).[24]

Between 1 and 3 percent of young men in Western countries have used AASs, including up to 12 percent of adolescents, while APEDs are used daily by one third of adults. AAS use is associated with cardiomyopathy (deterioration of the muscles of the heart), ischemic stroke, and liver toxicity, as well as side effects such as acne, hair loss, gynecomastia (male breast enlargement), hypogonadism (low testosterone levels), and infertility. They can also have serious psychological effects, including aggression and violence, hypomania, impulsivity, and depressive symptoms.[25] To the contrary, some people consider experiencing side effects a good sign that the steroids are working. As with other drugs of abuse, users can become dependent on them and are often at risk for other substance-use disorders.

Three patterns raise serious red flags in APED users: polypharmacy (simultaneous use of many drugs), body image disturbance, and disordered diet and exercise patterns.[26] Looking across several studies, 60 percent of AAS users also reported using nonsteroidal APEDs, while more than 90 percent used more than one AAS. They also combined steroids with central-nervous-system stimulants, thyroid hormones, ancillary agents, and nonsteroidal anabolic supplements. A unique part of this drug use is that APED users will borrow medicines designed to treat cancer, heart problems, or other ailments to manage side effects or boost the potency of their drug use. This cavalier approach to medication shows a worrying degree of comfort with pharmacology, with APED users basically acting as their own living laboratory experiment. Dr. Hildebrandt notes that many users view their polypharmacy as a chemical/pharmacological version of plastic surgery.

Lastly, diet and exercise disturbances commonly go hand-in-hand with APED use and include sticking to strict dietary regimens, obsessive-compulsive behaviors (such as an intense, excessive exercise plan), and feelings of guilt or loss of control with either eating or exercise. These things go hand-in-hand because achieving that lean, hypermuscular look requires not only APED use but also strict and extreme diets and exercise. Compounding the problem, extreme diets and exercise can exacerbate the negative effects of APED use. Increased caloric intake may lead to higher lipid levels or hyperglycemia, which can increase the risk of heart-related problems. High-calorie protein diets and supplements can also put pressure on kidneys and liver as they struggle to process the excess protein.

ROID RAGE

In June 2007, professional wrestler Chris Benoit (aka the Canadian Crippler) murdered his wife and son in their Fayetteville, Georgia, home before hanging himself from a weight machine.[27] When the initial investigation uncovered several prescription drugs, including anabolic steroids, in the home, speculation arose that Mr. Benoit may have been under the influence of a "roid rage," although untreated concussions were also suggested as playing a role. Toxicology reports later revealed that Mr. Benoit had injected himself with testosterone and taken two prescription drugs, hydrocodone (a narcotic painkiller) and Xanax (an antianxiety drug), but there were no illegal drugs or anabolic steroids in his system. While the levels of hydrocodone and Xanax in his urine were not abnormally high, the levels of testosterone were nearly ten times the top of the normal range.[28] Dr. Kris Sperry, the chief medical examiner of Georgia, noted, however, that these results were not sufficient to draw conclusions about possible "roid rage," pointing out that "an elevation of this ratio does not necessarily translate to something abnormal in a person's behavior. There is conflicting scientific data as to whether or not testosterone leads to any mental disorders or violent outbursts."

Nearly two years later, Dr. Phil Astin, Mr. Benoit's personal doctor, was sentenced to ten years in prison for illegally prescribing painkillers and other drugs.[29]

Body Checking. Given the different body ideals that some men (lean and muscular) and women (extremely thin) are striving for, it comes as no surprise that the way that men body check can also differ from women.[30] While women may look for cellulite on their thighs, men might test the hardness of their biceps. Likewise, while women might weigh themselves frequently for weight loss, men may compulsively check their body fat percentage. Indeed, the most common types of body checking endorsed by men are: "I check the hardness of my muscles to ensure that I have not lost any bulk," "I look at my abdominal muscles (six-pack) in the mirror," "I compare my overall leanness or muscle definition to others," and "I compare the size of my chest muscles with others."[31] In men with classic anorexia nervosa, the body checking is much the same as in women, such as checking the size of wrists or thighs or measuring size by the fit of clothes.

Muscle Dysmorphia. As discussed previously, cultural ideals for male body types have changed over the years. Media imagery can play a powerful role in propagating these trends and influencing men's perceptions of their own bodies.[32] When young men are presented with images of idealized male bodies preselected for being extremely muscular and attractive (in comparison to neutral images), afterward they tend to have greater levels of body dissatisfaction.

This cultural trend toward a desire for simultaneous increase in muscularity and decrease in body fat, when taken to the extreme, can manifest as muscle dysmorphia, which was originally called "reverse anorexia."[33] Men with muscle dysmorphia are preoccupied with being lean and muscular, have negative beliefs about their body, and may avoid or be anxious about their bodies, all of which can interfere with social, occupational, or other important areas of functioning.[34] So these men who are normal size, or even more muscular than average, may believe that they look "puny" or "small," which drives them toward strict dieting, intense workouts, or AAS use to achieve their elusive muscular ideal.[35] They may also feel intense anxiety and shame about showing their body in public and resort to wearing baggy clothing to hide what they perceive to be inadequate muscularity. Men with muscle dysmorphia report more areas of concern on their body, are more likely to lift weights or perform other exercise excessively, are more likely to diet and to have poorer scores on quality-of-life measures, are more likely to report a suicide attempt, are more likely to have abused AASs, and are more likely to have substance-use disorders or eating disorders than men with other forms of body dysmorphic disorder (a disorder in which someone is concerned and preoccupied with a perceived defect of his or her physical features).[36]

In a survey of 237 male weightlifters between the ages of eighteen and seventy-two, the "dysmorphic" group reported a number of very concerning behaviors, including the highest levels of quantity-frequency of exercise, supplement use, AAS-HGH use, and bulimic symptoms (including vomiting and laxative use to lose weight).[37] They also reported very high body dissatisfaction, obsessive-compulsive symptoms, and frequent tanning and body-hair removal. This same pattern holds among illicit APED users, with about 10 percent of them having muscle dysmorphia and a more severe drug use profile.[38]

When men try to simultaneously lose weight and increase muscularity, they often pursue extreme dieting in the form of consuming many small high-protein, low-carb meals per day, alternating cycles of weight gain and weight loss, or following a ketogenic diet. How these behaviors relate to eating disorders remains a mystery. We do not know whether these patterns are gateways into traditional eating disorders, or if this is a variant that simply exists on the periphery of the classic disorders. What we do know is that they are associated with psychological features that are shared with eating disorders (e.g., body dissatisfaction and body image distortion), and they pose considerable health risks, including increased body fat, renal changes, and elevated blood lipids and blood pressure.

Todd's story vividly illustrates how disordered behavior can have roots in childhood and far-reaching effects well into adult life.

I was always the skinnier, athletic kid when I was younger. But when I hit seventh grade, my metabolism didn't seem as fast . . . I started to get chubby and I didn't like it. Also, it seemed like my friends could eat anything they wanted and stay naturally lean. They were also natural athletes. That wasn't me . . . I had to work for it. So, I first started to look into how to work out and eat healthy. I wanted to get in shape and be leaner, be at top shape . . . the best I could be. But I not only wanted to be leaner, more defined, and more muscular, I wanted my performance enhanced. I wanted to jump higher, run faster. I had a friend who was going through the same thing, and we pushed each other with our diet and exercise. But I didn't compete with him—I always competed with myself. I enjoyed pushing myself to new limits.

I naturally tend to get obsessive and compulsive about whatever I throw myself into. I also like control. So when I started exercising and eating healthier, I learned all I could about it and really took it seriously . . . but I was unhealthy at first. I didn't know what I was doing and took it to an extreme. At twelve or thirteen, when I wanted to lose weight and get lean, I talked with the wrestlers who knew about how to cut weight. I also talked with my football friends who knew about lifting and getting lean. I started lifting weights, running, doing plyometrics, and playing basketball every day. I would do abs before bed at night. I also started eating less, cutting out all fats. People thought it was excessive, though they never worried. But I found I didn't have energy and couldn't build muscle, and I wanted to build muscle most of all.

I went to a high school that valued being big. Our school was known for football, and most of my friends were bigger. Some of them dabbled with steroids; for boys, doing steroids at my school was the equivalent of taking diet pills for girls. I never did them. I thought it was cheating and was scared about the side effects. I was the "good kid" in school. I was a peer counselor and involved in all sorts of campus clubs and activities. But because I played basketball, I had a hard time getting big—there was just too much cardio. To get bigger and stronger, I scaled back on the cardio and gained weight, going from one hundred fifty-five to one hundred eighty pounds just because I was curious to know what it felt like to be bigger, to have bigger muscles. I think this is an innate desire of most guys who work out, at least initially during adolescence.

By the time I left for college, I was one hundred eighty-five pounds. I was still training hard and eating really clean. I never ate dessert and cut out carbs. Then a nasty combination of events occurred that pushed me over the edge. First, the transition during college was incredibly hard for me. I felt like I had no control over my life. Also, I found out that my girlfriend of two years had cheated on me with my best friend. I was sick of being the "nice guy" and having people take advantage of me. The sense of lack of control I felt at the time played a huge role in my focus on changing my body. I was so messed up emotionally that I thought, "What the f***, if ever I'm going to do it, now's the time to go all in!" By that I meant to get as big as I could (muscle-wise) and get as strong as I could—to reach my upper limit.

This drove me to take steroids. I had something I could focus on and control when I otherwise felt out of control. As with anything, I went all in with it . . . working out daily and exercising one or two times per day. Eating a ton to gain muscle. With a friend, I first took 4-Androstene. Then I did one cycle of steroids, which had immediate and big effects. I went from one eighty-five to two fifteen in just two months. It felt so good working out; there's immediate reinforcement. You see your strength go up with almost every workout, and you get what we call "the pump": your muscles get tighter and enlarged, you get veiny . . . it feels really good. I also became the big guy at the gym. And guys appreciated that. They started approaching me more, asking me questions about how I worked out, what I ate, etc. You know, women hear, "Oh wow, you're so thin." For guys, it's "Oh wow, you're bigger." You definitely get reinforcement for getting big in that environment. It also gave me a sense of power. If you are in a situation, someone will think twice before messing with you.

Why did I stop? I realized it was not for me. I just wasn't myself . . . I became an angry, volatile person and couldn't control my anger. I would get in stupid fights with people, and I hated not having control of my emotions. It was painful! The steroids and routine really took a toll on me emotionally. It really was such a weird point in life that it is tough to even think about. I only did the steroids for three months, so I didn't have any physical side effects, but the psychological side effects scared the crap out of me, and that's what helped me stop. I got off the steroids right away, but it took a couple years for me to mentally recover and to finally get to be okay and accepting of my natural body type . . . to not be so obsessive with the gym and so "clean" with my eating. I used to hate eating out because I couldn't control what was in my food. But I'm much more flexible with that now. I've learned to work with my body type. I still like to push my body every day, but I want to live a long life, be happy and stable, and I don't want to have to take a bunch of supplements or work out three times per day. Getting into my career helped me get over that . . . I had a new passion and identity. I have more things I enjoy now, which helps balance things out and put into perspective what's important in life. I have other things that make me feel good about myself.

FORMER BRITISH DEPUTY PRIME MINISTER
DISCUSSES BULIMIA

In April 2008, John Prescott, the former deputy prime minister of the United Kingdom, revealed to the public that he had been suffering from bulimia nervosa since the 1980s. As a seventy-year-old man with diabetes, Prescott does not fit the bulimia stereotype, which was one of his motivations in discussing his disorder.

His bulimia began in the early 1980s while in the shadow cabinet, although it was not until the Labour Party came into power in 1987 that his symptoms worsened. He took refuge from his sixteen- to eighteen-hour workdays in food. He found comfort in feeling full and experienced a "weird kind of pleasure in vomiting and feeling relieved." Although he concealed his bulimia from the public, his wife recognized the disorder and encouraged him to seek help in 1991. He was still suffering in 1997 when he became deputy prime minister. Though Prescott suffered from bulimia for ten years, he remained silent because of the shame he felt at being a high-profile figure with the disorder. He stated that it was "difficult as a man like me to admit that I suffered from bulimia—the doctors told me that it was probably due to stress." His goals in sharing his experience were to destigmatize the disease, to encourage others to seek help, and also to show that bulimia can affect people other than young women.[39]

Obstacles to Seeking Treatment
Dr. Hildebrandt cites three critical obstacles that prevent men from seeking treatment for their eating disorders: stigma, sexuality, and access.

Stigma works on several levels. The broad-based belief that eating disorders are the domain of women may keep men from admitting or even recognizing that they have an eating disorder. Men also like to solve problems on their own and may be reluctant to seek professional help accordingly. Clinicians can inadvertently send men further underground if they are not receptive when men reach out for care. An insensitive remark about a "woman's disorder" or a quick dismissal of an eating disorder from the diagnostic possibilities because of preconceived notions about who suffers from eating disorders can cause a male patient to slip back into his shell and retreat into his eating disorder. Although family members might also be slow to recognize eating disorders in men, more commonly, I see family members who are aware and concerned, but who reach roadblocks with professionals who don't step up to the plate and follow through with appropriate referrals.

Sexuality is the second barrier. The widely held misperception that eating disorders in men reflect their sexual preference might make men think that, if they admit to an eating disorder, this may raise questions about their sexuality, which can make some men uncomfortable. The bottom line is, eating disorders don't really care about sexual orientation; they are equal opportunity afflictions.

Lastly, Dr. Hildebrandt highlights access to treatment as an important barrier. Many facilities treat only women with eating disorders or fail to provide programming tailored to male patients. It is not uncommon for a man to be the only representative of his gender in a treatment program or support group. This does not mean that it can't work; in fact, mixed-sex groups can be highly effective, but not all men are comfortable being the only guy in the room. As men with eating disorders are coming out of the shadows, we are seeing more and more programs evolving that cater to the specific needs of men seeking treatment.

AWARENESS AND ACTION

This exercise is about consciousness raising. If you're a woman, go to the store and buy a men's health magazine. If you're a man, go to the store and buy a women's magazine. Be prepared for what you are going to see and read. If you're in a relationship and are heterosexual, consider doing this together as a couple and talking about it. If you're in a relationship and are homosexual, think about doing it with your partner with a magazine targeting the opposite sex. Page through the magazine and talk about the images and messages you see. What are the ideals they are putting forward and telling the opposite sex that they need to strive for? Are these things that you think are important in someone of the opposite sex (regardless of your sexual orientation)? How do you imagine someone of the opposite sex would feel after reading this magazine? Would they measure up? Would you spend your money on this magazine? The answers to these questions can give you more insight into the impact of these publications on esteem. They can also provide you with insight into your children's behavior. Are you comfortable with your children reading these things? Think about how you can inoculate them against these messages and turn their attention to more worthwhile and self-affirming topics.

CHAPTER 5

The Changing Context of Eating Disorders

Parts of this chapter may be hard to read. If you have an eating disorder and you find numbers triggering, you might want to monitor whether you are getting stuck on figures rather than grasping the big picture. I have included some staggering statistics about our toxic food and activity environment because it provides important background for our understanding of the changing landscape of eating disorders. Our world has changed enormously in ways we never predicted. I think back on the futuristic cartoon *The Jetsons*, in which life was fully automated and food was hyperprocessed. The Jetson family had a treadmill that George and Astro ran on regularly, but none of the characters was challenged by the consequences of the biological collision of decreased energy expenditure and increased intake of highly processed foods. The rest of us have not been so lucky.

To contextualize the changing landscape of eating disorders, we need to address issues ranging from the global to the cellular. To understand the emergence of anorexia nervosa, bulimia nervosa, BED, and other eating disorders in midlife, we need to place them in the context of global and local trends in diet, physical activity, and media. This approach will help address how obesity and eating disorders can coexist not only in Western cultures but across the globe. We then have to look under the microscope to understand how genetics and biology influence how we respond to these trends. Only by merging our understanding of the global context with an appreciation of individualized biological response to environmental changes can we truly understand the reasons behind the demographic shift of eating disorders.

Not a day passes that we don't hear about the "war on obesity" or the "fight against childhood obesity." Michelle Obama, Bill Clinton, Jamie Oliver, Charles Barkley, and countless others have joined the celebrity army to fight this enemy that is waging war on our society. But how did we get here and when did we declare war?

Although eating disorders are about so much more than weight, weight is still an important component. The old guard firmly believed that weight regulation came down to a simple equation: calories consumed versus calories burned. In principle, although these remain the fundamental elements of the equation, there are many more factors involved in weight regulation than we initially believed. We have all heard overweight people claim that they hardly eat anything and still put on weight. Perhaps there's a flicker of disbelief in your mind when you hear someone say that because you adhere to the "calories in equals calories out" doctrine. But we are not all the same, not all calories are the same, and the answer is not that straightforward. First, let's evaluate the basic equation and outline what we already know about how our society has shifted in terms of its two core variables.

Calories In

When I was a child, we ate breakfast and dinner at home as a family and went out to eat maybe once or twice a week, at the most. When I visited my relatives in Germany for the first time, I realized that eating dinner together across three generations was the central activity of the family (and neighborhood) every evening; everything happened around the dinner table. Kids might have come and gone after the meal, but the family table remained the hub throughout the evening, where parents, grandparents, visiting relatives, and neighbors were gathered. Dinner took hours, and the conversation flowed in all directions. If more visitors stopped by, another cup of coffee was poured and another slice of cake was distributed, and they joined in the conversation. Dinner was family and community combined.

Today, on average, Americans eat a meal outside the home about every other day, and about half their annual food expenditures are in restaurants.[1] According to the 2006–08 American Time Use Survey (ATUS), the average American spends only sixty-seven minutes per day engaged in primary eating and drinking (i.e., this was the main activity) across all meals and snacks.[2] This is certainly a far cry from the leisurely meal and evening's entertainment in my German relatives' home. In 1970, Americans spent about six billion dollars on fast food; in 2000, they spent more than one hundred ten billion. They now spend more money on fast food than on higher education, personal computers, computer software, or new cars.[3]

The impact of this shift on the quality of food we consume is very apparent. "When people eat out they tend to make poorer nutritional choices," says Lisa Mancino, a food economist for the United States Department of Agriculture quoted in 2011 in the *Orlando Sentinel*, "partly because people often associate eating out as a special occasion, or a time to splurge—even if eating out has become a routine."[4] She expands her observations to indicate that eating one meal away from home each week translates to about two extra pounds a year.

Most Americans are no longer aware of what an appropriate portion size is. Neither the food pyramid nor the new MyPlate[5] graphic can remedy that, especially when up against the onslaught of portion distortion brought on by Big Food and Big Beverage. Born out of free-market competition and the American desire to get the most value for your dollar, fast-food chains competed with each other to provide more caloric bang for your buck. Even though the following statistics seem to be repeated over and over, they still don't seem to shock people into action. An average 1950s fast-food meal consisted of a

1.6-ounce hamburger, 2.4 ounces of French fries, and a 7-ounce soft drink, totaling 598 calories, 23 grams of fat, and 716 milligrams of sodium. Today's average meal has ballooned to an 8-ounce hamburger, 7 ounces of French fries, and a 32-ounce soft drink, bringing the total to a whopping 1,580 calories, 68 grams of fat, and 1,405 milligrams of sodium![6]

The "Get Government Out of My Kitchen" movement will say that it is our personal responsibility to stop eating when we're full, but that simplistic statement ignores an enormously dense psychology behind both economics and appetite. First, 54 percent of Americans will eat until their plate is clean.[7] Whether this has to do with our grandmothers' voices in our heads or childhood admonishments to remember the "starving children in Africa" is unclear, but we rely on that external cue (an empty plate) rather than signals from our stomach to our brain (satiety cues) to tell us when to stop eating. On the economic side, "I paid for that food, doggone it, so I'm going to eat it all up" is another incentive to down every last bite: Food not eaten is seen as money wasted. Together, those two forces are more powerful than the impact of any appetite hormone that might encourage us to exhibit free will and say, "Stop eating now." Accordingly, as portion sizes have increased, so has our consumption and so, inevitably, have our waistlines.

This transformation has led to two outcomes that are particularly relevant to midlife eating disorders. First, it has increased the discrepancy between most people's body sizes and the societal thin ideal. As we get larger, we are further and further away from the ideals set forth in the media; they become even less attainable. So body dissatisfaction becomes ubiquitous, and many people either engage in sequential self-defeating cycles of dieting or simply give up. Second, the transformation has blurred the line between overeating and binge eating. The definition of a binge as an "unusually large amount of food by social comparison" has shifted and is no longer clear. A standard fast-food meal today might have been considered a binge in the past, but now, by social comparison, it is normal.

Portion distortion has hit not only restaurants but also our homes. Cookbooks have also supersized their recipes. Over the past seventy years, calories per serving of home-cooked meals have gone from 168.8 to 436.9 calories, which represents a 63 percent increase in calories per serving. Of the eighteen recipes published in all seven editions of the *Joy of Cooking* over this time period, seventeen increased in calories per serving.[8] This can be attributed partly to a jump in total calories per recipe, but also to larger portion sizes. For example, the chicken gumbo recipe went from yielding fourteen servings of 228 calories each in the 1936 edition, to ten servings of 576 calories each in the 2006 version.[9]

Finally, if you're one of those people who is distracted by fellow moviegoers chomping on popcorn during the film, brace yourself. In the 1950s, a movie theater serving of popcorn was just three cups. So an irritable moviegoer could anticipate the first few minutes of the show being a problem, followed by silence through the middle and end of the film. Today, the average serving size is sixteen cups, which can lead to chomping distractions right up through the middle of the movie. If we continue to escalate at the same rate, be prepared to watch more movies in the comfort and silence of your living room!

Taste Bud Abuse: Sugar Onslaught

Another insidious factor keeping our ability to regulate intake off-kilter is sugar. According to the United States Department of Agriculture, the average American consumes 297 cups of sugar every year. This is way, way above recommendations from the American Heart Association, which say that people who follow a 2,200-calorie diet should limit sugar intake to about 68 cups yearly.[10]

Let's do a breakdown starting with what has become public enemy number one: sugar-sweetened beverages. To be clear, in general, I am a firm believer in staying away from labeling foods as "good" or "bad." However, sugar-sweetened beverages, at least in the quantity that they are consumed in the United States, come closest (next to trans fats) to challenging my principles. Every ounce of regular soda contains about 1 teaspoon of sugar. Now imagine eating the same amount of sugar straight from a teaspoon: a 12-ounce can has 12 teaspoons of sugar (192 calories), a 20-ounce bottle has 19 teaspoons of sugar (304 calories), a 32-ounce bottle has 31 teaspoons of sugar (496 calories), and a 64-ounce container has 62 teaspoons of sugar (992 calories)![11] Carbonated soda and fruit drinks are the major sources of added sugar in the American diet, and these numbers make it clear why.[12]

In my book *Crave: Why You Binge Eat and How to Stop*, I deal extensively with what I call stealth sugars. Few people are aware of just how frequently sugar is added to their foods. *U.S. News & World Report* lists foods that contain unexpectedly high amounts of sugar, including baked beans (15 grams of added sugar per cup), regular or low-fat ketchup (as much as 40 grams per serving), reduced-calorie French dressing (58 grams per serving), canned peaches in heavy syrup (28 grams per serving), and jelly beans (19.6 grams per 10 large pieces).[13] One of the effects of these added sugars is that they make other unadulterated food taste bland. Your brain becomes accustomed to ubiquitous hyper-sweetness, to the point where you feel compelled to add Splenda or another sweetener to fresh summer strawberries. Sadly, sweets, desserts, soft drinks, and alcoholic beverages account for nearly 25 percent of all calories consumed by Americans, while healthy fruits and vegetables make up only 10 percent of caloric intake in the U.S. diet.[14]

The Nonfoods We Eat
We simply have no idea what the full impact of all the nonfood substances added to our food is on our ability to regulate our appetite or weight. These days, reading ingredient labels is more

challenging than studying for an organic chemistry exam. The following ingredients were unearthed by the company BodyEcology and represent a partial list of a chemical soup of preservatives, flavorings, and additives that can be found in the artificial flavoring in a strawberry "milkshake." Ask yourself, without investigating, would you willingly put a teaspoon of any of these in your mouth? Your child's mouth? Your grandchild's mouth?

> Amyl acetate, amyl butyrate, amyl valerate, anethol, anisyl formate, benzyl acetate, benzyl isobutyrate, butyric acid, cinnamyl isobutyrate, cinnamyl valerate, cognac essential oil, diacetyl, dipropyl ketone, ethyl butyrate, ethyl cinnamate, ethyl heptanoate, ethyl lactate, ethyl methylphenylglycidate, ethyl nitrate, ethyl propionate, ethyl valerate, heliotropin, hydroxphenyl-2-butanone (10% solution to alcohol), a-ionone, isobutyl anthranilate, and isobutyl butrate.[15]

In addition, whether any of these compounds influence eating disorders, or how they do so, is simply unknown.

THE ALL-AMERICAN CHAMELEON FOOD: CORN

We are corn. Medical journalist Sanjay Gupta, M.D., turned to University of California, Berkeley, plant biologist Todd Dawson for a hair analysis. A full 69 percent of the carbon in Dr. Gupta's hair came from corn. Illustrating that we are what we eat, Dr. Dawson commented, "We are like corn chips walking." After Dr. Dawson had spent three months in Italy, his own hair content was a mere 5 percent corn, illustrating dramatically how much more corn-y Americans are than Europeans.[16] More than 25 percent of the approximately forty-five thousand items in American supermarkets contain corn, including disposable diapers, toothpaste, batteries, and even magazine covers. In the United States, most meat is derived from corn, as chickens, turkeys, pigs, and cows are fed a corn-based diet, and fish aren't escaping this new diet trend, as even farm-raised salmon are fed this staple.[17] Given that dietary diversity is key to overall health, as well as a predictor of positive outcome for anorexia nervosa, the ubiquity of hidden corn is an obstacle we need to surmount.

Eating Patterns

Living in the United States, you don't have to have an eating disorder to have dysregulated eating; in fact, dysregulated eating is the norm. Lack of predictable, regular mealtimes is an insidious backdrop to midlife eating disorders, as eating disorders are more likely to gain a foothold when habitual eating and noneating times are not being followed.

What we say is not necessarily what we do. Although 93 percent of Americans have heard their mothers tell them that breakfast is an important meal for an overall healthful diet, 56 percent still don't eat breakfast every day, according to a 2009 survey from Food Insight.[18]

We also eat anytime and anyplace. Malls, sports stadiums, movie theaters, roadside rest stops, twenty-four-hour convenience stores, shoe stores, electronics stores, department stores, even gyms and health clubs—the food checkout ambush is everywhere. The absurdity is mind-boggling at times. Americans can't work out at the gym without thinking they have to replenish their glycogen stores with a high-cal smoothie before they leave the health club. We can't hit up the mall without thinking we need a snack to fuel our shopping adventure. We can't buy books without succumbing to the tempting smell of a muffin and a cappuccino. We are constantly, and I mean constantly, bombarded by food cues. There is no food "downtime." Paradoxically, we don't cook anymore. So it's no wonder that a recent survey gauging societal norms in thirty-four countries revealed that Americans spend the least amount of time cooking per day: just thirty minutes.[19] Although we may be riveted by TV shows that pit wannabe celebrity chefs against each other with a basket of ingredients in a challenge to create a novel meal, most of us would be paralyzed by this task, unable to repurpose a stalk of raw broccoli if our lives depended on it. The Institute of Food Technologists (IFT) in an annual survey reports that fewer than one third of American households make meals from scratch. And even though you might find three quarters of Americans around the dinner table at home, almost half of the food they're serving at that table is pre-prepared at restaurants, supermarkets, or fast-food outlets, according to the IFT.[20]

The 1950s marked a revolution in the kitchen. The advent of prepackaged meals accompanied women's entry into the workforce. Enter the microwave, fast-food chains, and an eat-on-the-go mentality and we have today's trends.[21] In fact, television shows and cooking magazines tout partial recipes in which you include some raw ingredients but build the meal around processed foods. Sandra Lee has made a cottage industry out of semi-home-cooked meals (70 percent processed, 30 percent from scratch).[22] How is it that we have time to watch hours of cooking shows on several food networks yet don't have time to cook for ourselves?

The relevance of all of this to midlife eating disorders is vast. Everything about our food environment is dysregulated: what we eat, where we eat, how we eat, and when we eat. Each facet of disequilibrium paves the way for the development of disordered eating behaviors, whether it be the complete lack of a satiety compass brought on by portion distortion and nonnutritive flavor enhancers, or an extreme reaction to these forces leading to outright food rejection.

Clearly, Western society is set up for overconsumption, but it is also set up for underconsumption, and these lures coexist and are mutually reinforcing. Returning to the insidious interplay of big industries, Big Food, Big Beverage, and Big Diet positively feed off each other's successes and failures. Diet, low-fat, nonfat, artificially sweetened options exist for almost every food. These products convey the false message that "it's okay to eat more" of a particular product because it is reduced in some ingredient that is judged to be excessive or "bad" for you (i.e., sugar, fat, salt). (This of course sidesteps the question of why the "bad for you" options are marketed in the first place.) Unfortunate side effects of this strategy exist for the individual that once again benefit the industry. When an individual who is embarking on an eating episode opts for a low-fat version of a food, this triggers a decision cascade in the person's mind that results in the thought "Since it's low-fat, I can eat more of it." She then ends up eating virtually the same amount of the sugar, fat, or salt she would have eaten had she eaten a smaller amount of the regular variety, plus . . . drumroll . . . Big Diet makes more money because she purchases two instead of one! And, the "diet" variety is more expensive.

The extent to which we are biological victims of the Big Industries becomes infuriating when you take a bird's-eye view. We are simply biologically incapable of self-regulating in a completely dysregulated world. Our bodies were not made to resist the ubiquitous torture wreaked upon us by alternating overconsumption and dieting, which results in lifetime cycles of yo-yo dieting.

Calories Out

Now that we've covered calories in, let's deal with calories out. America is out of step with other countries when it comes to physical activity.[23] A 2010 study by a nonprofit organization called America On the Move tracked the number of steps taken by 1,136 adults around the United States who wore pedometers for two days and compared the results to similar studies in Switzerland, Australia, and Japan. Americans, on average, took 5,117 steps per day, far short of the benchmarks in Western Australia (9,695 steps), Switzerland (9,650 steps) and Japan (7,168 steps). The standard definition of "sedentary" is taking fewer than 5,000 steps per day, and in this study American men averaged 5,340 steps and women only 4,912.[24]

In her continuing inquiry into changes in American lifestyle, Tara Parker-Pope of the *New York Times* highlighted changes in the nature of our jobs as one culprit.[25] Reporting on a study conducted of occupation-related physical activity,[26] she recounted that jobs requiring moderate physical activity, which accounted for 50 percent of the labor market in 1960, have plummeted to just 20 percent. The remaining 80 percent of jobs are sedentary or require only light activity. The shift in on-the-job movement translates to an average decrease of about 120 to 140 calories a day in physical activity, which is a close match with the steady weight gain in the United States over the past five decades.

The workplace isn't the only place we're not moving. A poll of 6,329 individuals revealed that Americans spend 7.7 hours a day being sedentary, which could include working, studying, driving, or being transfixed by the TV or another screen.[27] Late adolescents, people over sixty, and women were among the most sedentary groups. This behavior is bad for our bodies and bad for our metabolism. We were designed for movement, so it is no wonder that we are seeing a rise in workplace-related injuries when we are depriving our bodies of the physical activity they need to stay in top form. Many people wonder why they are still not able to maintain a healthy weight even if they are going to the gym three times a week. Well, the energy expended in those three hours at the gym doesn't balance out the metabolic molasses that characterizes our sedentary lifestyle the other one hundred sixty-five hours per week.

Martha, age fifty-four, went to the gym three times a week

and was a regular at twice-weekly step aerobics classes. Smack in the middle of menopause, she lamented that she was still putting on weight and gaining girth around the middle, despite this religious workout routine. What Martha did not take into consideration was how much of the rest of her life was spent completely motionless. The Centers for Disease Control and Prevention's 2008 *Physical Activity Guidelines for Americans*[28] recommends that adults engage in one hundred fifty minutes of moderate-intensity aerobic activity (the equivalent of brisk walking) per week, plus muscle-strengthening activities on two or more days per week that target all the major muscle groups. Regardless of how much moderate-to-vigorous exercise people do over the course of a week, taking more breaks from sitting throughout the day is associated with having a smaller waist circumference, lower BMI, and lower triglyceride and plasma glucose levels.[29] So, to be healthy, you don't necessarily have to become an ultra-marathoner, but you do need to give your body movement throughout the day. It's somewhat ironic that so much of our entrepreneurial spirit over the past several decades has been directed toward making life more convenient, and now we have to actively combat that convenience with motivated physical activity in order not to succumb to the health consequences of inactivity.

The Impact of the "Nutrition Transition" on Eating Disorders Globally

The United States no longer corners the market on eating disorders or obesity. In fact, the rest of the world is catching up at breakneck speed. The term "nutrition transition" was coined to explain the rapid and dramatic shifts in diet and physical activity patterns that have occurred around the world in recent decades as societies undergo economic growth, urbanization, and industrialization.[30] But as diets have become more "Westernized" (higher in fat, cholesterol, added sugar, animal food products, and processed foods, and lower in fiber) and levels of physical activity have declined (via changes in leisure activities, automation, transportation, and work), there has been a parallel rise globally in obesity and other nutrition-related noncommunicable diseases, such as cardiovascular disease, diabetes, cancer, and eating disorders.

The rise in obesity is not limited to high-income countries and is occurring in countries as diverse as Mexico, Egypt, Brazil, and China. The rate at which obesity is increasing in many lower- and middle-income developing countries in Asia, North Africa, and Latin America is two to five times faster than in higher-income countries such as the United States; and the burden of obesity is falling squarely on the shoulders of the poorest people in the population.

In many developing countries, malnutrition and obesity coexist—sometimes in the same household. When obesity is paired with imported Western media, body dissatisfaction ensues. The gulf between actual body size and desired body size widens and can be the impetus for extreme weight-control behaviors, triggering anorexia and bulimia nervosa in all age groups. The irony of coexisting malnutrition and eating disorders is a painful reality as the nutrition transition parallels the export and adoption of Western media-driven thin ideals.

The propagation of the Western media's thin ideal, and the parallel male lean and muscular ideal, has long been suspected to play a role in the development of disordered eating behavior and eating disorders around the world. Studies have been conducted in all corners of the globe and in various cultural contexts to try to understand how and why this pernicious export can influence the development of disordered eating. Young girls surveyed in the 1980s in their native Greece had a lower prevalence of anorexia nervosa than young Greek girls living in Germany,[31] which was attributed to the radical changes in the social and cultural landscape experienced by the families of Greek migrant workers who relocated to Germany in the 1960s and 1970s, including greater exposure to Western thin ideals.

Perhaps the most groundbreaking work on the export of Western media and its impact on body dissatisfaction and eating disorders has been conducted by Anne Becker, M.D., Ph.D., Sc.M., and her team in Fiji. They documented an increase in disordered eating behaviors and attitudes in adolescent girls after television was introduced to the islands in 1995. Even if girls didn't have direct media access, the fact that their peers did strongly influenced the extent to which they were affected by Western thin ideals, once again showing the powerful effect of social networks on influencing body dissatisfaction and disordered eating.[32]

Japan also has a long history of stringent standards for female beauty, focusing on features as far-ranging as skin tone and foot size, and has experienced an influx of Western advertising, fashion, and movies. Now women of all ages have increasingly turned to dieting to reach a thinner body standard, which has become equated with beauty and success in contemporary society. While the prevalence of overweight and obesity has grown dramatically in many parts of the world, adolescent and young adult women in Japan have actually gotten smaller! The average BMI of women aged fifteen to twenty-four decreased from 21.5 in 1960 (the equivalent of five feet five inches and one hundred twenty-nine pounds) to 20.5 in 1995 (the equivalent of five feet five inches and one hundred twenty-three pounds), raising concerns that increased dieting in this age group could be driving the rise of eating disorders.[33]

Christine C. Iijima Hall noted at the time that "Asian women [were] deluged with images of the perfect woman— tall, blonde, buxom, thin, with European facial features," and suggested that as Asian women are, by nature, farther from this Western ideal, they may be even more vulnerable to developing eating disorders as they judge themselves by a "European barometer." Western influence is evident in changing beauty regimens in Japan, where young women chase American ideals portrayed in the media through cosmetic surgery, chemical processing of hair, and tanning.[34]

The Japanese Health Ministry has spoken out due to concern that the number of young, skinny women has risen to troubling levels. A staggering 29 percent of Japanese women in their twenties are underweight (BMI <18.5). According to an ABC News report in 2012,[35] Yoko Saito from the health ministry's Movement to Improve National Health stated, "The women are not at risk of health problems yet, but we are making it a goal to bring the number down to twenty percent in the next decade." Saito explained that the government is treating diminishing waistlines as a national health issue, especially since the problem could affect fertility rates in a country that already has one of the lowest birth rates in the world. And this trend is not limited to youth.

Can exposure to Western thin ideals alone actually cause eating disorders? Or are there other factors at play? Part of the equation is how large the gulf is between a given native culture and these Western ideals. In a study of South Asian and Caucasian adolescents in the United Kingdom, the prevalence of bulimia nervosa was higher in South Asian girls (3.4 percent) than in Caucasian girls (0.6 percent). But somewhat surprisingly, higher scores (indicating greater risk) on eating attitudes tests were associated with those girls who had a more traditional cultural orientation (e.g., use of native South Asian language, dress, and food). So, having a foot in both cultures—especially when the native culture is quite different from the Western one—may put one at particular risk for developing an eating disorder.[36]

Culture also influences the face of eating disorders—not only regionally, but also across time. Several years ago, I was exploring Rome with Federica Tozzi, M.D., an Italian colleague who also does research on eating disorders. Having been raised Catholic and grown up playing the organ, I have an unquenchable fascination with visiting churches and cathedrals around the world. We stumbled upon a fairly nondescript church, but as always, I was compelled to check it out. The church was the Basilica of Santa Maria sopra Minerva, which houses the remains of Saint Catherine of Siena, joint patron saint of Italy along with Saint Francis of Assisi.

Born in Siena, Italy, around 1347, Caterina Benincasa was deeply affected by witnessing the death of several of her siblings. She had her first vision of Christ at an early age and vowed chastity at age seven. The curator at the church recounted stories of her life that sounded identical to what my colleague and I were accustomed to seeing in our clinical practices, but presented in a religious package rather than one of Western thin ideals. The curator explained that, despite her extensive travels, writing, and speaking, Catherine ate progressively less over the years, often subsisting only on Holy Communion. The clergy and sisters feared for her life, but Catherine claimed she was unable to eat. She described her lack of appetite as an illness, which has been labeled by others as *anorexia mirabilis* or "miraculous lack of appetite," referring to religiously motivated anorexia. Much like those who have the purging subtype of anorexia nervosa, she would regurgitate what she swallowed and reported severe stomach pains, which she incorporated into penance for her sins. With the exception of the religious explanatory model, Dr. Tozzi and I could find little difference between Saint Catherine's suffering and that of our contemporary patients.

Elsewhere, modern case studies of apparent anorexia nervosa among adolescent and young adult women in India, all of whom demonstrated classic food restriction and drastic weight loss, seemed to lack the body image distortion, desire for thinness, and fear of becoming fat necessary to meet Western diagnostic criteria for anorexia nervosa.[37] Likewise, "poverty, poor health, and low fecundity" in Korea and China, as well as dynamic social change, particularly with regard to roles and opportunities for women, may be playing a role in the rise of body dissatisfaction and disordered eating in those societies.[38]

No one expected to find cases of anorexia nervosa on the Caribbean island of Curaçao, where overweight is socially acceptable. But a review of medical records of the entire island revealed similar rates to Western countries. Exploring topics related to eating, body image, migration, and exposure to different cultures revealed that the women with anorexia nervosa, who were well-educated, high-income, and had spent time overseas, reported higher levels of perfectionism and anxiety, as well as greater influence on their eating patterns from family, peers, and modern fashion than women without eating disorders.[39] Those with eating disorders also expressed isolation and disconnection from the cultural norms in Curaçao, and a strong desire to belong, equating thinness with both success and belonging. These findings hark back to Anne Becker's work in Fiji, where her in-depth interviews revealed that young girls equated the Western thin ideal with their dream occupation of becoming a flight attendant, opening up opportunities for them to see the world. So clearly we're not just talking about appearance for appearance's sake, but a complete package of what the thin ideal symbolizes in terms of opportunities and aspirations.

How Metabolism, Brown Fat, and Sleep Affect Weight
Some individuals hold hard and fast to the rule that overweight or underweight simply reflects an imbalance in the "calories in equals calories out" equation. Some will say that any deviation from that fundamental equation defies the First Law of Thermodynamics. Others disagree.

Until now, we have been looking primarily at external environmental factors that influence eating behavior, physical activity, and weight regulation and dysregulation, but that is just part of the equation. There are also a number of individual biological factors that affect these dimensions. We know that a variety of genetic and environmental factors can interact with diet and lifestyle to influence who gains weight, who loses weight and keeps it off, who is able to maintain very low weight (as in anorexia nervosa), and who develops medical complications from obesity.

The humble laboratory mouse has come to the rescue numerous times to help us answer some of the basic questions about metabolism that form the foundation of our understanding of weight regulation. Until now, there has been a limitation to studies done using mouse models. Mice that are bred in laboratory settings are inbred, meaning they are the product of twenty or more generations of brother-sister mating to ensure that they maintain very specific traits, which are usually traits that predispose them to certain human diseases. For example, Black 6 mice have low bone density, develop age-related hearing loss, and are susceptible to diet-induced obesity, Type 2 diabetes, and atherosclerosis, while other strains of mice serve as excellent models for Type 1 diabetes, rheumatoid arthritis, leukemia, autism, and seizures. Mice called DBA/2J are teetotalers: They just don't like alcohol. BALB/c, by any other name, are scaredy-cat mice; they're afraid of everything.[40] This kind of uniformity is excellent for doing research on specific conditions that a mouse strain is prone to, but these inbred strains don't come close to representing the vast genetic diversity seen in the human population. To truly model the complexity of weight regulation, eating behavior, and physical activity in humans, we need mice that are as diverse as a cross section of people in the world.

In an effort to re-create the diversity of the human population, researchers at the University of North Carolina at Chapel Hill bred a new line of mice called the Collaborative Cross (CC) by using eight different founder strains including strains that were predisposed to the development of diabetes, obesity, and insulin resistance.[41] After generations and generations of cross-breeding, they ended up with a population of CC mice that reflect the breadth of human genetic diversity. The beauty of the breeding program is that, while the researchers do not know the exact genetic makeup of complex humans, they do know the exact genetic makeup of every CC mouse because they can trace the genes that got passed down at each cross all the way back to the genes of those original eight founder strains.

Under unrestricted conditions, the extent to which weight, activity, and body fat differed across the eight founder strains and 176 new lines of CC mice was mind-boggling. The mice weighed between 15.0 and 35.5 grams, and their body fat percentages ranged from 1.1 to 31.7 percent. These are whopping differences. Interestingly, body fat did not necessarily correlate with body weight; there were some low-weight but fat mice and some high-weight but lean mice. The researchers also studied physical activity (measured by running on a wheel), respiratory exchange ratio (a measure of energy utilization or "calories out"), food intake, and changes in body weight and body fat percentage in response to exercise. When given free access to a running wheel for twelve days, some CC mice hardly ran at all ("couch potatoes"), while others covered nearly twelve miles in a day ("half-marathon mice")! In addition, calories in and calories out were not neatly paired: Some mice ate a lot and ran very little, while others ate very little and ran a lot. The most enlightening observation was that exercise didn't affect all mice equally. After twelve days of running, although some mice showed the expected decreases in body fat, other mice actually had a higher body fat percentage than before exercising— despite being fed the same amount. The investigators do not yet know precisely what factors contribute to these differences, but it is clear that genetic factors play an enormous role in how individuals respond to variables like diet and exercise. And, obviously, the old adage about calories in equaling calories out is far too simplistic to account for the myriad processes that affect body weight regulation and dysregulation.

Another factor that makes the story more complex is that

not all fat is created equal. Humans actually store two types of fat, "white fat," which is what we have the most of, and "brown fat," which actually does have a bit of a brown hue because it is filled with mitochondria (the cell's "power plants").[42] We've known about brown fat for a long time. Infants and hibernating animals don't shiver; rather, they use brown fat to generate heat to keep them warm. Only recently have researchers discovered small amounts of brown fat in adults, mostly in the upper back, along the neck and shoulder, and down the spine. Women have more brown fat than men, and people who are older or overweight have less than their younger, thinner counterparts. So what does this mean for human metabolism?

A team of endocrinologists in Quebec exposed six healthy men to cold temperatures. The researchers controlled the environment and the temperature to keep shivering to a minimum (since shivering can burn calories) and measured the metabolic activity of the men's brown fat. The brown fat actually used white fat as a fuel source to generate heat to keep the participants warm, which increased the men's overall energy expenditure by an average of 80 percent.[43]

A second team of researchers from the Dana-Farber Cancer Institute, a teaching affiliate of the Harvard University Medical School, found that exercise actually generates another type of brown fat, which is found interspersed in white fat.[44] They discovered a new hormone, called irisin, that converts white fat to brown fat during exercise in mice. Since humans have an identical version of irisin, it's possible that some of the calories we burn during exercise, which incidentally are more than the calories needed to actually do the exercise itself, are burned during the process of converting white fat to brown fat. Since brown fat has superior calorie-burning properties, exercise might have longer-term benefits by making more brown fat that helps burn energy.

Sleep is also an issue. The prevalence of obesity in the

United States was 22.9 percent from 1988 to 1994 and rose to 30.5 percent by 1999 to 2000.[45] Over this same time period, the average amount of sleep per night reported by Americans decreased by approximately 1.5 to 2 hours. From 1950 to 1960, the most commonly reported sleep duration in the United States was 8.0 to 8.9 hours. However, the 2002 Sleep in America Poll indicates that, on average, adults in the United States reported sleeping just 6.9 hours per night.[46] Thus, as BMI has gone up, sleep has been going down. Just because two phenomena are correlated doesn't mean that once causes the other; however, given the number of bodily systems that are involved in both sleep and weight regulation, it was sensible to investigate this association.

A large national study explored the relationship between average number of hours of sleep per night and BMI and found that individuals between the ages of thirty-two and forty-nine who reported an average of six, five, and two to four hours of sleep per night were 27 percent, 60 percent, and 235 percent more likely to be obese than individuals who reported seven hours of sleep per night, respectively.[47]

Sleep and weight are related in many complex ways. Less sleep is associated with changes in hormone function and metabolism, which can decrease the sensation of satiety (fullness) and energy expenditure, and lead to increased hunger and food cravings.[48]

But how does sleep affect risk for eating disorders? Women who reported not getting enough sleep, sleeping poorly, having problems falling asleep, feeling sleepy during work or free time, and having disturbed sleep were significantly more likely to report binge eating, even after accounting for other factors such as age, obesity status, depression, and whether they were living with someone, all of which could interfere with sleep.[49] The nature of the association between sleep problems and binge eating is probably as complex as that between sleep problems and obesity. Sleep problems may lead to binge eating, binge eating may lead to sleep problems, or both sleep problems and binge eating may be the result of a third factor, such as stress in the environment, depression, or other biological factors. One compelling possibility is that many of the same metabolic and hormonal pathways may be involved in sleep, weight, and binge eating—and a single disruption in the pathway could interfere with all three.

Stress may also be a common factor underlying both sleep problems and binge eating, as it is a known culprit for both.[50] The hypothalamic-pituitary-adrenal (HPA) axis is the key hormonal pathway that regulates the body's stress response. Cortisol, our main stress hormone, is regulated by the HPA-axis, and when cortisol goes up, food intake increases in women.[51] Higher cortisol is also associated with more severe binge eating.[52] Intriguingly, high cortisol is also associated with less sleep.[53] So one way this could all tie together is that high cortisol could stimulate appetite and eating and increase the risk of developing binge eating.

Another variable to throw into the mix is night eating (see Chapter 2). Around 11 percent of women who report binge eating also indulge in night eating, and 20 percent of those who night eat also report binge eating.[54] Interestingly, there is considerable overlap in the genetic factors that contribute to these two behaviors, suggesting that there may be some joint biological pathway that influences binge eating and night eating. The relationship between dysregulated sleeping and dysregulated eating may be even more tight than we initially believed.

As we struggle to get enough sleep, and to have our children and grandchildren get enough sleep, these results support the argument for adequate sleep being an essential component for overall health and well-being, including weight regulation and prevention of disordered eating.

Placing Blame Where Blame Is Due

The forces that influence the changing landscape of eating disorders are vast and require us to use every lens—from telescope on the global issues to microscope on the cellular issues. The tragedy of the situation is that we continue to blame the individual . . . for being overweight, for losing control of eating, for losing control of dieting. We spend billions of dollars, spend countless hours doing research, and spend enormous amounts of money on health care because we are addressing the problem on the level of the individual. We come up with new types of bariatric surgery, seek new drug targets for obesity and anorexia, develop and test new therapies, all to help individuals resist an environment that they are biologically incapable of resisting. In no way am I saying that we should not be developing these interventions, but our efforts directed toward the individual are dwarfed by the opposing forces of the Big Industries. More research on public health policy is required to level the playing field to give our interventions a chance and to give individuals hope.

Imagine this challenge. You have been treated for cocaine addiction, yet when you surf through your television stations, you come across three different "Cocaine Channels." Each one shows tempting drug-related cues twenty-four hours a day. Or you've spent hundreds of dollars on smoking cessation programs, and when you buy a bottle of water at the airport at the checkout the clerk asks you, "Would you like a delicious cigarette to go with that?" Or, after successful treatment for heroin addiction, you drive past billboard after billboard of drug paraphernalia luring you into the next heroin drive-through that is just 1.5 miles away. Or, after rehab for alcoholism, you go shopping for clothes at the mall, and the food court is replaced with the "Bar Court" and you had to navigate the gauntlet of the Irish Pub, the Scotch Bar, the Wine Cellar. Well, these absurd scenarios differ very little biologically from what the individual with BED experiences when driving down the highway seeing billboard after billboard advertising fast-food restaurants, or when walking through the food court at the mall. They also differ little from the individual with anorexia nervosa walking into a "health food" store and seeing supplement after supplement promising rapid and sustained weight loss. The losers here are the individuals. The winners are the Big Industries. I'm not talking about nanny-state policies, but I am talking about leveling the playing field and limiting the extent to which industries can market products and create environments that we are biologically and psychologically unable to defend ourselves against.

Big Beverage and Big Food create a binge-friendly environment. And our sedentary, convenience-oriented lifestyle makes going to the restroom during the day practically our only required physical activity. At times, it can feel like a Sisyphean task to create change on a macro level, but if we keep whittling away at that which is under our control, we can at least create local change that may ripple upward. The bottom line is that we don't have to buy into any of this—either conceptually or by reaching into our pockets. Being aware is the first step; developing a resistance plan comes next.

AWARENESS AND ACTION

One way to combat the environment is to establish and maintain regular sleep, eating, and exercise routines and identify forces that interrupt them. Now, if you have babies or young children who still wake up in the middle of the night, some of this is out of your control. If you're a perimenopausal woman who wakes up multiple times during the night swimming in sweat, you too have challenges to regularity (but talk with your physician about this—there are options!). Regardless of these uncontrollable factors, identify your daily anchors. What are the events that are consistent time anchors in your day? For example, I have a strong morning anchor. Breakfast, coffee, and the newspaper (yes, the old-fashioned paper kind) form the anchor of every day. Even when I am on the road, I re-create this anchor by eschewing breakfast meetings and making sure I have this single focal point to maintain a consistent pattern across days.

For a week, use your smartphone or your computer or jot down on paper the time you wake up, the time you go to sleep, and the times you eat each day. At the end of the week try to see if you have any reliable behavioral anchors and evaluate the extent to which your patterns are regular or all over the map. If you are fairly regular, great, you're already on the right path. If you see a more chaotic pattern, address how you can define a workable anchor for yourself and try to implement that for the following week—whether it be eating lunch at noon every day, taking a break and a brief walk at ten A.M., walking the dog at seven P.M.—something to provide a consistent and predictable event every day to start to establish a more regular pattern. Also note your sleep duration and see where you stand relative to the statistics in this chapter. It is enormously more difficult to make positive changes in your life if you are sleep-deprived.

CHAPTER 6

Genes and Environment at Any Age

For decades, the causes of eating disorders have been misunderstood. We know now that they are caused by a confluence of genetic and environmental factors, but our challenge is making that information widely known. Unfortunately, it is much harder to remove misconceptions from people's minds than to plant new, accurate information. Let's take a classic, frightening example. In 1999, British gastroenterologist Dr. Andrew Wakefield and his colleagues reported a relationship between the measles, mumps, and rubella (MMR) vaccine and autism.[1] This report put parents around the world in a panic and led many to withhold potentially life-saving vaccinations from their infants, starting an antivaccine fervor in the United States. The sheer number of times the words *vaccination* and *autism* were used together in the newspaper, on television, and on the radio only further cemented them as connected in people's minds.

What people didn't realize, however, was that this finding was just a correlation. Although the two things occurred at the same time, one did not necessarily cause the other. In fact, the study was later declared to be fraudulent and was retracted from the scientific literature![2]

Even as scientists reiterate that there is no connection between the MMR vaccine and autism, many celebrities continue to support Wakefield's claims and place doubt in the public's mind.[3] For example, model and actress Jenny McCarthy has stoked the fires and advocated the need to reassess all vaccines and their ingredients because they could be harmful to children. Her Generation Rescue campaign has ingrained this questioning attitude into its list of statutes.[4] This continued attention has encouraged media outlets, such as the Huffington Post, to discuss the MMR vaccine "controversy," placing the general public into a confused and confusing scientific and political environment.

Such misinformation can be seriously dangerous to public health. That study remained in the literature for twelve years before its retraction and, during the heyday of vaccination fears, diseases that had been eradicated started rearing their heads again. In the United States, outbreaks of whooping cough (pertussis) and mumps came back on the scene, and daycare centers and doctors' offices became high-risk venues in under-vaccinated areas—all because of misinformation based on fraudulent research.

This intentional foray into vaccines and autism illustrates the important point that misinformation about health can be extremely damaging. Although not blemished by fraudulent data, blatant misconceptions and stereotypes have also seriously hampered the eating disorders field. As captured eloquently by Gloria Steinem, "The first problem for all of us, men and women, is not to learn, but to unlearn."[5]

We've already examined the myth about who suffers from eating disorders; now we'll deal with what causes them. Historically, the family (and, most often, mothers) have been blamed for causing many disorders in their children. For decades, it was believed that certain types of families were more likely to have children who developed eating disorders. In a book published in 1978, Salvador Minuchin, a psychiatrist originally from Argentina, described families with an anorexic child as enmeshed, overprotective, rigid, and unable to resolve conflict.[6] It seems that, whenever medicine can't explain an illness, a parent is blamed.

We also saw this with autism before it was recognized as

a neurodevelopmental disorder, as Bruno Bettelheim in 1967 described the "refrigerator mother" whose coldness and aloofness clearly resulted in her child's autism.[7] Similarly, in 1948 Frieda Fromm-Reichmann[8] blamed schizophrenia on the "schizophrenogenic mother," who induced psychosis with conflicting rejecting and overprotective behavior. Later, the whole family was blamed for having communication styles that put the emerging patient into unresolvable double binds.[9]

Even today, you may encounter ill-informed clinicians who make damaging offhand comments like "no wonder she has anorexia—look at her mother," or "if my mother were that controlling, I'd have anorexia too." As with autism and vaccines, the more frequently these concepts are paired in people's minds—regardless of accuracy—the more they become indelible. Overprotectiveness does not cause anorexia nervosa, but having a child with anorexia nervosa sure can make you overprotective. They had it all backward. Sure, family functioning can affect eating disorders, but eating disorders also have a deep and widespread impact on family functioning—including relationships with parents, partners, and children.

The second misconception that has impeded the understanding of eating disorders is that they are a choice—that the person with anorexia nervosa simply chooses not to eat, or the person with BED chooses to binge, or the person with bulimia nervosa chooses to vomit. Concepts such as choice and willpower have clouded our ability to understand the forces that drive these behaviors. These erroneous beliefs have persisted, in part, due to inaccurate empathy. All of the features associated with eating disorders fall along a continuum of normal behavior. Most people have gone on a diet at some point in their lives—but few have starved to the point of anorexia. Most people have overeaten—but fewer have experienced true binges with a sense of being out of control. Most people have vomited—but few have self-induced vomiting for weight loss, or to undo the effects of a binge. Most people have experienced body dissatisfaction or a desire to be thinner—but far fewer have spiraled into a pit of complete self-loathing of their body.

Yet the fact that we have some personal experience with "light" versions of these core features lures us into believing that we can understand what causes them and how to stop them. We believe that, if we can choose to stop eating after a second helping, then other people should be able to stop a binge. Or, if we can stop dieting and go back to regular eating after we lose five pounds, then people with anorexia nervosa should be able to choose to go back to regular eating. With other psychiatric disorders like schizophrenia, the continuum conundrum doesn't exist in quite the same way. It's not as if we've all had a few minor hallucinations that allow us to empathize with hearing voices inside our head or believing that we're receiving messages from the television. The break between the reality of someone with schizophrenia and our reality is more clear-cut. With eating disorders, however, inaccurate empathy leads to misunderstanding.

Another reason for the persistence of misunderstanding is what I call the "tyranny of face validity." Eating disorders can all be conveniently rationalized by sociocultural explanations that quite simply make too darned much sense. This face validity has deeply hindered progress in the field and prevented partners and families from developing a deep understanding of their loved one's disorder. For example, the sociocultural theory of anorexia nervosa focuses on ubiquitous exposure to the Western thin ideal and posits that women with anorexia nervosa internalize this ideal and seek to attain the desired model figure presented in the tabloids or on television. This simple explanation makes perfect sense to the onlooker: you see a skinny model in a magazine, you hear your girlfriend say she hates her body and wants to lose weight, you make a connection, and voilà, the sociocultural model has face validity. What you miss is the critical inflection point where the model weighs one hundred fifteen pounds and your girlfriend starves down to seventy. That is far, far beyond what any fashion magazine would ever showcase.

On the other end of the spectrum, you hear and read about the obesity epidemic, ballooning portion sizes, and the decline of family meals, and you think, of course, these societal factors are what causes someone to binge eat. The model has face validity. What you miss is that there is nothing in that model that predicts the sense of loss of control, or the intense urge to binge, or the shame and distress that ensue after the binge is over.

Together, these myths, misconceptions, and misplaced empathy have impeded research, interfered with detection and treatment, and created enormous misunderstanding in families and couples about what eating disorders are, what causes them, and why they can be so intractable to intervention.

Race, Ethnicity, and Midlife Eating Disorders
Another entrenched myth about eating disorders is that they affect primarily Caucasian individuals. This is yet another misconception that has stood in the way of accurate detection and treatment. In fact, some of our work on race, ethnicity, and eating disorders may have inadvertently backfired. The data are clear: African-American and Hispanic women do suffer from eating disorders, although as mentioned before, there is some suggestion that anorexia nervosa may be slightly less prevalent in African-American women than Caucasian women.[10] The critical piece of information is that women from diverse racial and ethnic groups are less likely to seek treatment and to be referred for treatment than Caucasian women.[11]

The detection piece is most likely due to eating disorders being off the radar screen of clinicians, but the treatment-seeking piece is also a worry. In many minority populations, eating disorders are highly stigmatized—even more so than other mental illnesses. This can be a powerful inhibitor of reaching out for treatment. Dr. Mae Lynn Reyes-Rodríguez at the University of North Carolina is working to break down the barriers to treatment seeking by reaching out to community organizations and clinics where Latino families go for health care. Also keenly aware that the majority of our treatments for eating disorders were developed for and tested on Caucasian patients, she is adapting eating disorder treatments to be culturally appropriate for Latino patients. By attending to cultural factors such as *familismo*, or placing a strong emphasis on family relationships, by including family members even in the treatment process of adult patients, and by dealing directly with issues such as stigma, religion, documentation, and immigration stress, she is embedding the treatment into the constellation of culturally relevant ideals and challenges that Latinos in the United States are facing. Moreover, she is delivering these treatments in community centers, which helps to destigmatize the disorders and demystify the treatment process.

One of the explanations that has been forwarded for the lower rates of anorexia nervosa in African-American women is that they have greater tolerance for a broader range of body shapes and sizes so there is less pressure to diet down to a cultural ideal, thereby exposing fewer women to unhealthy weight-loss practices. While this may be true, there may be some inadvertent side effects of this interpretation. An African-American woman came in for an evaluation for BED, which in her case was marked by extreme body dissatisfaction. She had been suffering for years, and when asked why she was seeking an evaluation now, she reported, "I have hesitated to come in because being a black woman, I am supposed to be happy with my large body. Everyone says that we black women are happy in our bodies no matter what the size. I wondered what was wrong with me, there wasn't just something wrong with my eating, I wasn't being a good enough black woman because I didn't like my body. Then I finally said, forget it, forget all of these shoulds, something is wrong and I need help!"

Genes Load the Gun and Environment Pulls the Trigger
We now know that relatives of people with anorexia and bulimia nervosa have more than ten times the risk of developing
an eating disorder at some point in their lives, compared with
relatives of people without eating disorders—but it is not always
the same eating disorder.[12] Family patterns can include an aunt
with bulimia, an uncle with anorexia nervosa, and a number of
people throughout the family tree with various degrees of
EDNOS. In other words, eating disorders do not "breed true." In
many ways, this makes perfect sense since, as we have seen in
Chapter 2, the boundaries between and across eating disorders
in an individual can be quite fluid over time. BED, however, may
be somewhat distinctive, as relatives of individuals with binge
eating disorder are more than twice as likely to develop the disorder themselves than relatives of individuals without BED.[13]

Strategies exist to help tease out whether genes or environmental factors are the dominant culprits for why something
runs in families. Large-scale studies of twins are an excellent
way to determine which plays a weightier role. Twin studies
use large samples, sometimes in the tens of thousands, of
identical and fraternal twins to catalog how often both members of a twin pair have the disorder of interest. Since identical
twins share 100 percent of their genome (i.e., they are virtual
clones) and fraternal twins share only 50 percent of their genome, if both members of identical pairs are more likely to
have the disorder than both members of fraternal pairs, then
there is a better chance that genes are involved. Figure 3 illustrates why genes are likely to be involved in the familial pattern
seen in anorexia nervosa, but not in the purchasing of a Chevy.

Figure 3 compares the role of genes in the familial pattern
of anorexia nervosa and in the purchasing of a Chevy. It illustrates two hypothetical twin populations to illustrate the concept. Pairs of emoticons that are the same shade represent
identical twins, and those that are different shades represent
fraternal twins. Any emoticon on the right side of the figure with

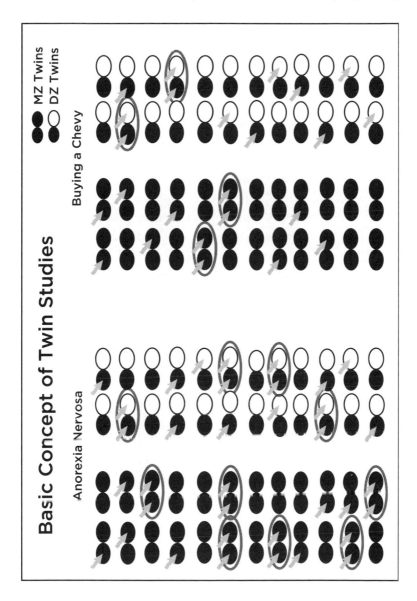

an arrow is a Chevy buyer and those on the left with an arrow have anorexia nervosa. A circle around a pair means that both members of the pair either bought a Chevy or had anorexia (i.e., they are concordant).

For Chevy buying, pairs of identical twins and fraternal twins are equally likely to both buy Chevys: about 25 percent of the time, both members of both types of twins buy the same brand of car (concordant for Chevy buying). On the left side of the graphic, both members of identical twin pairs are much more likely to have anorexia nervosa than both members of fraternal twin pairs (concordant for anorexia). Since those identical twins are genetically identical, while the fraternal twins are not, this is decent evidence that genes may be involved in anorexia, but not in Chevy buying.

We can also get more sophisticated with statistics and calculate the heritability of a disorder, which tells you what percentage of liability to that disorder is due to genetic effects, and several studies have done this for eating disorders. If we apply those statistics to Figure 3, the heritability of purchasing a Chevy would be 0 percent, meaning that environment is the key factor in picking a car. In contrast, the heritability of anorexia nervosa would be more like 60 percent, which corresponds with what has actually been found in scientific studies.

This type of twin study on eating disorders has been conducted in several countries around the world. One of the limitations of this body of literature is that most of these have been conducted primarily in Caucasian populations of European ancestry, so we simply don't know if the same numbers hold in more diverse populations. With that caveat in mind, the heritability of anorexia nervosa has been estimated to be between 22 percent and 88 percent, the heritability of bulimia nervosa between 28 percent and 83 percent,[14] and the heritability of BED between 40 percent and 57 percent.[15] Although these numbers are high, and on par with other mental illnesses such as bipolar disorder and schizophrenia, an important thing to note is that the heritability estimates are not 100 percent, which means that environment is also playing an important role. The current understanding is that genetic factors work in concert with environmental stressors to influence risk for eating disorders.

When we say that genes are involved in eating disorders, what do we actually mean? First, we don't mean that there is one anorexia nervosa gene or one bulimia nervosa gene or one BED gene. We know that these are complex disorders that are influenced by the interaction of multiple genetic and environmental factors. So, if you wake up in the morning and read a headline that says ANOREXIA NERVOSA GENE FOUND, you know the journalist (or at least the person who wrote the title) didn't understand the science. A heritability estimate also does not imply what percentage of cases are genetic: A 50 percent heritability estimate does not mean that 50 percent of the cases of bulimia nervosa in the world are genetic cases and 50 percent are environmental cases. These are complex statistics that focus on variance in a population and simply reflect what proportion of the liability of developing an eating disorder is due to genetic factors.

Most critically, the influence of genetic factors in no way signals destiny. These are not like single gene disorders where, if you have a specific mutation in a specific gene, there is a 100 percent chance that you will develop the disorder. Nor are they like Huntington's disease, where offspring of someone with the disease have a fifty-fifty chance of developing Huntington's themselves. Genes do not signal destiny for traits as complicated as eating disorders. In fact, you could have several eating disorder risk genes but never develop an eating disorder if, for example, you never go on your first diet.

Basically, our "risk soup" contains four ingredients: risk genes, protective genes, risk environments, and protective environments. Of course, actual risk is more complicated than this, and many of these factors can interact, but for most intents and purposes, understanding these four ingredients will get you

pretty far in understanding your risk. We're born with an as-
sortment of risk and protective genes from our biological mothers and fathers, and there is not much that can be done about
this basic genetic makeup.

It's important to remember what genes do. They don't give
you anorexia, or make you impulsive. Biologically, genes just
code for proteins and then downstream, things get very complicated. So the genes are the scaffolding, while throughout our
development, the environment flings all sorts of arrows our
way, as well as numerous lifelines and buffers. It is the critical
combination of genetic risk and protective factors, plus environmental risk and protective factors, that ultimately deter-
mines whether we ever develop an eating disorder. At the core,
genes load the gun, but environment pulls the trigger.

So the question remains, if the genes are there since conception, what has changed in the environment that is leading
to more midlife eating disorders?

EMBRACING COMPLEXITY

Humans prefer all or nothing, black or white, certainty over
probability. However, science rarely affords us the opportunity
for this kind of clarity. Our understanding of biology and genetics is rapidly unfolding, but with each new discovery, we seem
to uncover another layer of complexity. Genetics is like the
universe within: vast and complicated, with hidden dimensions,
no outer limits, black holes, bosons, and yet-to-be-discovered
phenomena that are lurking beyond our awareness but are actively influencing how our genes are expressed. For this reason,
we refer to eating disorders as "complex traits," and to understand them, we have to reach beyond our desire for simplicity
and embrace complexity. For a definition of a complex trait, we
turn to the executive summary of a report from a panel of ex-

perts who met at the National Institutes of Health on December 10–11, 1997, at a workshop entitled The Genetic Architecture of Complex Traits.[16]

> Most genetic traits of interest in populations of humans and other organisms are determined by many factors, including genetic and environmental components, *which interact in often unpredictable ways.*
>
> For such complex traits, the whole is not only greater than the sum of its parts, it may be *different from the sum of its parts.*
>
> Thus, complex traits have a genetic architecture that consists of all of the genetic and environmental factors that contribute to the trait, as well as their *magnitude and their interactions.*

This concise summary illustrates how far beyond "genes load the gun, and environment pulls the trigger" we need to go in order to truly grasp the complexity of risk for eating disorders. Although our risk soup still fundamentally comprises those four ingredients of risk and protective genes and risk and protective environmental factors, this definition highlights that there is no simple algorithm that can predict who will develop a disorder. The principle of unpredictability, and the fact that the whole can be different from the sum of its parts, reflect not only the magnitude of our lack of understanding, but also the impact of seemingly random forces on human outcomes. We are biologically complex, and we are bombarded by an incalculable number of environmental forces every day, which are impossible to capture in any prediction equation. Somewhere between our desire for simplicity and feeling dwarfed by unfathomable intricacy is the stance of embracing complexity that we must adopt to understand the risk of developing eating disorders.

Midlife Triggers

Between adolescence and midlife, your genes don't change (although how they are expressed can change), but what does differ to some extent are the environmental triggers that can set off, reignite, or sustain eating disorders at different stages of life. Although just about any major stressor could trigger an underlying predisposition to an eating disorder, there are a few that are making a recurrent appearance in midlife women and men who are presenting for treatment. Some of these represent reignited old traumas or experiences that were associated with disordered eating in the past. Some of them are unique to adulthood and may trigger an eating disorder for the first time, or retrigger a dormant eating disorder in a new way. Here are the most common ones that we have encountered in the clinic.

Infidelity. Liza never thought it would happen to her. She had counseled countless friends whose husbands had strayed, but she and David had been together for almost twenty-five years—they had met in high school, they had started dating right away, and everyone knew that they would always be together. They had recently been planning a vacation and doing Internet searches for unique destinations. David had identified some cool places on the coast, but Liza couldn't remember the names. He was out on a bike ride, so she decided to just check his browser's history. As she scrolled down the list, Liza found some vacation spots and some work-related websites, but then she found a whole list of Internet sex sites. This wasn't just porn; they were interactive sex sites. She started shaking and thought she was going to throw up. Nobody else used this computer. David was betraying her with Internet sex. Her first thought was that she wanted to kill him. Her second thought was to wonder whether it was her fault. Her interest in sex had gone down precipitously during perimenopause: Was this his way of getting back at her for not wanting to have sex as often? She ran downstairs, downed an entire half-gallon of ice cream, then went to the bathroom and vomited everything up. She hadn't done that in thirty years.

Don Baucom, Ph.D., Distinguished Professor of Psychology at the University of North Carolina at Chapel Hill and an expert on couple interactions, states, "Finding out that your partner was unfaithful creates a deeply visceral sense of shock, disgust, and disbelief. All that you believe about your partner and your relationship is destroyed. Your sense of control is gone, and there is nothing safe left to cling to. Most people experience a desperate urge to escape from the horror and feel better immediately. For some people, that sought-after comfort comes in the form of an out-of-control binge that might bring momentary relief or distraction from the interpersonal nightmare. Of course, it is destined to fail beyond the moment, because the road to recovery from an affair is a long and complex process that does not start in the refrigerator."

It is not just the aggrieved party who can be at risk for disordered eating.

Dawn thought she was happily married and had always believed that once you make that lifelong commitment, no one else can open your heart. But then she was working at the community garden one afternoon and found herself staring at a young man who, from across the field, made her heart flutter. She worked her way over to his side of the garden just to get a closer look, and when he turned around to smile, she felt like she was back in high school with an adolescent crush. Dawn found herself chatting him up, and the conversation flowed easily from one topic to another. They worked side by side in the garden for two hours, and she heard herself asking him out for coffee afterward. Had she really done that? Did that invitation just come out of her mouth? He was at least fifteen years younger than she! That coffee was the first step toward a sordid affair.

Although their connection was positively electric, Dawn was always painfully aware of the fifteen years that separated them. Was he really attracted to her older body? How could she compete with women his age? She joined a gym, started doing hot yoga, went on a diet, and became determined to lose ten pounds. The ten pounds became twenty, and she became increasingly convinced that the way to keep their affair alive was to slim down.

He started worrying about her health and found that whatever spark they had felt was fading. He worried that it was his fault that Dawn was losing so much weight and decided that the dishonesty of their affair was driving her down this dangerous path. He broke things off, which devastated her. She was convinced it was because of her age and her weight. Dawn buried her heartbreak in further weight loss until she reached a dangerously low weight and was rushed to the emergency room by her husband, who had found her unconscious on the bathroom floor.

Dr. Baucom relates how infidelity in midlife can be a major stressor on both the relationship level and the individual level and can be a prominent trigger for midlife eating disorders. "'If only—if only I were younger; if only I were petite, if only I could make myself more appealing, people would love me and wouldn't leave me,'" he says. "Affairs often hurt everyone involved, even the person who initiates them. They often feel bad about themselves for getting involved since the majority of people, even those who have affairs, agree that affairs are wrong. And when they don't work out, people often feel like failures in the realm of love and intimacy. So why starve yourself in response to having an affair? For Dawn, there were lots of reasons—to be thinner and more appealing, to distract herself from the loss of her lover with a concrete goal of losing weight, and to punish herself for this exciting yet loathsome affair when she already had a loving husband."

Divorce. Even the most civil of divorce proceedings can keep you off-kilter for years—and the messy ones can create total upheaval. Divorce can trigger disordered eating in several ways. For Ashanda, it was the stress and anxiety. With every e-mail that came in from her attorney or her ex-husband's attorney, every piece of divorce-related mail, every time either of the attorneys' numbers popped up on caller ID, she would flush and tremble. After these encounters, she would stay stressed for hours with no appetite whatsoever. She was one of those people for whom anxiety eliminated appetite. Ashanda lost twenty pounds during the course of her divorce proceedings.

Camille, however, had the opposite reaction to the stress of divorce. She would go to the mailbox, find a letter from her husband's attorney, and dig into a box of cookies while staring at the letter, thinking it might open itself. Every familiar number on caller ID, every e-mail, every letter triggered a binge. The stress of divorce can disorder your eating either way—and the more contentious, the more extreme.

Sometimes there is even a delayed response. You may have girded your loins and trudged bravely through divorce proceedings, only to have signs of deep stress emerge much later. Martha, who started to binge eat a year after her divorce, recounted, "As the shock of my divorce wears off and the trauma sinks in a bit, I have come to a realization. I was able to get through the initial shock and pain by vacationing and connecting with friends, but what I know I need now is to regroup, sit still long enough to experience the pain, and get my health back. My head says I am not stressed and that I'm doing great. I willed this belief and convinced myself of this—yet my body is screaming otherwise. I've gained twenty pounds and had numerous health issues, most of which I believe are connected to my post-divorce stress level. My head is pushing, pushing, pushing, and my body is putting on the brakes, saying, 'Whoa, pay attention to me, we've got some work to do here to get past this.'"

Even months after the divorce, new divorce-related triggers can set in, such as loneliness or the fear of being back on the dating circuit, which can lead to engaging in unhealthy weight-control practices aimed at looking a certain way to be "marketable," such as going on the "divorce diet."

Empty Nest. Jay and Monica had raised four children. For nearly two decades, their lives revolved around work and the kids. Every night was a tight orchestration of who was driving who where, who was helping with which homework, who was cooking, and who was signing permission slips. They complained about never having a minute to themselves, yet they loved every minute of parenting. As one child after the other went off to college, Monica started planning for the inevitable. She had been talking with her friends about their empty-nest experiences and didn't want to be caught unprepared. She joined a storytelling group, began teaching adult Bible study, and started a beginners' ballroom dance class.

Jay didn't think empty-nest syndrome was something that hit men, so he made no preparations. He was just looking forward to spending more evenings watching sports. But after the last child was away at school, and Monica was off in the evenings for her activities, he started feeling the emptiness. At first, Jay reveled in *Monday Night Football*, but not alone: He was joined by a few beers and a bag of chips, sometimes two. Then it got worse, and he added ice cream, sandwiches, and cookies. Soon it became the food he looked forward to, rather than the football. If Monica canceled one of her activities, and he didn't have privacy to binge, Jay became annoyed and irritable and started binge eating in his car while driving around. One night, he spilled chili in the car while eating and driving and, although he tried to clean it up, Monica smelled it the next morning and asked him about it. He was ashamed to admit that the kids' leaving had affected him so much, but Jay sought treatment for BED, and they began looking for things they could do together in the evenings as a couple.

As illustrated by Jay, empty-nest syndrome isn't for moms only. Men too can be hit or even blindsided by the last child's walking out the door. There are both procedural and emotional factors associated with an empty nest that can be triggers for disordered eating. Many couples claim that their attention to healthy food, regular eating times, and nutrition in general is greater when the kids are still around. Once they leave, comments such as "It's not worth the trouble just for the two of us," or "We'll just grab something," are commonly heard. Even families who placed considerable emphasis on family meals can slip and fail to emphasize "couple meals" once the children are gone. Not only is this bad for your health and nutrition, but it probably isn't good for your relationship either. Coming together at mealtime is as important for couple maintenance as it is for family maintenance. Continuing to prioritize nutrition and the sharing of meals can help with the procedural part of the empty-nest–eating disorders equation.

The emotional component of empty-nest syndrome is more challenging. People change during the twenty years it takes to raise children and launch them into their futures. Often, those changes go undetected in the day-to-day flurry of running the family and emerge as an unexpected—and sometimes unpleasant—surprise when the children leave. "This is not the person I married" is often heard once couples are faced with just each other day in and day out. Simultaneously, you have lost one of your major day-to-day roles, namely parenting. Of course, you are still a mother or father, but you no longer have that all day, every-day, hour-to-hour sense of being needed, for everything from changing a diaper to finding the car keys. Daily visual and physical contact with your children gets reduced to phone calls or Skype and a few visits a year. If you're a physical family, your daily quota of physical affection goes down. All of these factors can cause someone to turn to food or, alternatively, starvation for comfort. For some, the mediating variable is mood. Children leaving home, along with problems reorienting to being a couple, can lead to feelings of low mood or depression, which themselves can influence eating behavior. Binge eating can be a way of self-medicating low mood or a way of counteracting boredom or emptiness.

Troubled Nest. Although an empty nest can be a stressor, trouble in the nest can be even worse. Dealing with adolescent or young adult children who are facing medical illnesses, psychiatric problems, legal issues, unemployment, or their own relationship or financial woes can be unexpected and serious stressors on an adult. The strain of dealing with adult children can be compounded if paired with responsibility for aging parents. The emotional crush between the two generations can be a stress from which escape seems impossible; even the most caring person can become overwhelmed with responsibility. One common side effect of overcommitted responsibility is not taking time for your own health and well-being. Eating on the run, no exercise, and no relaxation can amplify into binge eating or purging for stress relief, or self-starvation in an attempt to feel in control of something in your life. There is no more important time to care for yourself than when you are responsible for others. Otherwise, both your caregiving and your own health will suffer.

Bounce-Back Children. You did your job, got the kids through high school and college, and then, due to the economic downturn, there was no job for them on the other end. You waited and waited to hear whether any of those interviews yielded offers, but as March and then April came around, the dreaded call came. "Mom, can I come back home and live with you guys until I find a job?" You may have been planning a vacation, a downsizing, or more romantic nights alone, but all of a sudden, one of the little birdies is bouncing back. If you haven't set any ground rules, grocery bills go back up, sleep gets interrupted, rooms of the house get taken over, the car gets commandeered, and laundry and cooking duties revert to previous high levels, all of which can lead to unexpected stress that can trigger or retrigger an eating disorder.

As much as you love them, there comes a time when it becomes increasingly difficult to share a space with your children. As more and more families are facing this new midlife transition time, it is clear that terms have to be negotiated before the kids return home: It is, after all, still your house. Terms can include rent, a contribution to grocery bills, laundry and cleaning assistance, curfews, limits on noise after certain hours, negotiation for sharing the television or the car, and a frank discussion of any limits regarding sex, alcohol, and drugs in the home. Remember, you don't want to make it too comfortable, or there will be no incentive for your child to get a job and a place of his or her own.

Retirement. After years of waking to the alarm clock and being gainfully employed, the unstructured days and nights associated with retirement can be a shock to the system. If you haven't planned for the long hours with no demands on you, you can feel quite lost and directionless. To prevent yourself from turning to food to fill the empty hours, you may need to build structure into your retirement routine. This can guard against boredom and aid in maintaining a strong sense of meaning and belonging in your life.

Unemployment and Financial Concerns. More than at any other time in my professional career, adults suffering from disordered eating are identifying finances as triggers and perpetuators of their eating problems. The ways in which this manifests vary widely. Elisa, who had a history of bulimia nervosa, and her husband both lost their jobs. They went from a comfortable living, being able to afford lots of fresh, unprocessed foods to help maintain healthy eating habits, to having to make difficult decisions about weekly budgets as their financial situation crumbled. Even though they tried to preserve their eating style, eventually the weekly food budget had to come on the chopping block. Organic foods were replaced with cheaper bulk foods bought at a wholesale store. The pantry was suddenly filled with large boxes of cereal (a former binge food), mac and cheese, and other bulk products they could get on sale. Fruits were limited to apples, bananas, and, occasionally in the summer, and when affordable, grapes.

For the first time in her life, Elisa was thinking about how to put food on the table, rather than what food to put on the table—and soon something inside her rebelled. Home alone, unemployed, and bored, Elisa resented having to buy this "crap food." In her anger and desperation, she found herself, once again, bingeing on old favorites. Once her husband realized that food was disappearing, she felt doubly guilty for eating through the family's food budget.

Unemployment or underemployment, boredom, and the hit to self-esteem that comes with being poor are all triggers of our times. And financial triggers aren't limited to only those in lower income ranges. Previously financially comfortable individuals who have found their nest eggs eroded may also turn to food or starvation in desperation as they see worst-case financial scenarios unfolding before them—worse outcomes than they could ever have planned for and ones with far-reaching implications for their current lifestyle, their children's education, and their retirement.

Illness or Surgery. A subgroup of patients point to an illness as the catalyst of a midlife eating disorder. For some, an illness might have forced them to restrict certain foods, or not eat at certain times, which became the first step toward more extreme restricting. Patients with severe gastric reflux may start cutting out foods to reduce symptoms that, when taken to an extreme, can lead to severe weight loss. Gallbladder surgery, diabetes, celiac disease, and irritable bowel syndrome can all be initial triggers for the development of restrictive eating. Another often observed pattern is when patients take their doctors' orders to an unhealthy extreme. A recommendation to watch their cholesterol, lose some weight, or monitor their blood pressure may at first lead to healthy weight control behaviors but later morph into more extreme actions. The old adage "If a little bit of something is good, then a lot is better" just doesn't hold in this situation. When accurate vigilance becomes an obsessive preoccupation with cholesterol levels or a blood pressure reading, then the pursuit of health starts interfering with overall well-being.

Surgery can also be a trigger, and one surgery in particular that is having an unexpected effect of sparking eating disorders is bariatric surgery. We reported on a case of an individual developing anorexia nervosa after gastric bypass surgery as far back as 1999, prior to which there had been few case reports.[17] But the procedure was relatively uncommon then. Joanna Marino and colleagues suggest that the emergence of an eating disorder after bariatric surgery is a rare, but clinically concerning, phenomenon.[18] Our recent experience suggests that the numbers may be on the rise, although the reasons for this are not entirely clear. One possibility is that presurgical screening is either absent or missing the warning signs. Patients may fear that they will be turned down for surgery if they reveal a history of an eating disorder and, therefore, withhold this information. This is unfortunate, as failure to disclose these details may simply rob them of the opportunity to get adequate nutritional and psychological support before, during, and after surgery. A second possibility is that something about the surgery itself acts as a biological, mechanical, or psychological trigger for an eating disorder. As described by Dr. Maureen Dymek-Valentine, a clinical psychologist who has worked extensively with individuals undergoing bariatric surgery at both the University of Chicago and the University of North Carolina, "Many of these patients have long histories of dieting, which has always ended in frustration and weight regain. They have dealt with low self-esteem and social stigma. Then they have surgery. Presto—no more hunger, no more cravings, and food actually seems unappetizing! They think, 'Wow, I don't know how long this will last, so I am going to take advantage of it . . . I will skip this meal, and the next, because

I am not hungry.' They lose weight and feel great. Then, before they're even aware, they become fearful of eating even small amounts because they're terrified of going back to the dreadful past. They have been there, and they refuse to go back." This pattern underscores the critical importance of post-surgical monitoring and the value of rapid referral for treatment if these potentially dangerous patterns set in.

Yet another trap is when patients develop or continue to suffer from BED after surgery. Studies have shown that bariatric surgery can curtail binge eating;[19] however, it is far from a universal cure. Dr. Christine Peat, a clinical psychologist who works with bariatric surgery patients, clarifies that "many patients forget that bariatric surgery isn't tantamount to behavior change, which is necessary for the successful treatment of binge eating. For a lot of folks, binge eating remits during the 'honeymoon phase' right after surgery, but will recur after the weight loss has plateaued and they begin to experience an increase in stressors. They don't realize that their struggle with weight wasn't just about what they ate and how frequently—it also resulted from factors like emotional/stress eating and using food as a way to cope with life's stressors. It's absolutely critical that patients develop healthy coping skills after surgery to help prevent the (re)emergence of binge eating and, thereby, potentially undoing all the benefits of surgery."

Perimenopause. Perimenopause has been described as female purgatory. Also called the "menopausal transition," it is the period of time when a woman's body transitions from being fertile and having regular menstrual cycles and ovulation, up to the age of permanent infertility or menopause. You don't know how long perimenopause will last or how symptoms will affect you. One patient asked me when she could stop carrying emergency tampons around in her purse, and the truth is that it is wise to keep that stash around for quite a while. Officially, once you've gone twelve consecutive months without a menstrual period, you've reached menopause. If you go for six months and menstruate again . . . then you reset that clock.

Symptoms of perimenopause can include sleep problems, hot flashes (aka "power surges"), night sweats, vaginal dryness, mood symptoms, concentration difficulties, and changes in menstrual patterns with increasing irregularity. Every woman goes through this period differently, and since many of our mothers didn't talk about such things, we don't know what to expect.

Dr. Samantha Meltzer-Brody, director of the University of North Carolina Women's Mood Disorders Clinic, shares that we do know a few things that can help you prepare for perimenopause. First, the average age of menopause onset in the United States is fifty, and most women will experience at least four years of some sort of perimenopausal symptoms, with a range of one to ten years. This can start in your fifties, forties, or even thirties, and the degree of symptoms can vary in both type and severity. For example, some women will be most bothered by changes in sleep, mood, and concentration—finding themselves wide awake and unable to sleep at night, followed by feeling highly irritable the next day. Other women report feeling overwhelmed by hot flashes, described as a sudden onset of intense heat, sweating, and discomfort that makes one want to immediately strip off all clothing, regardless of the setting. Dr. Meltzer-Brody adds that some women report distressing changes in libido (or at least changes that are distressing to their partners). Many describe a decrease in sexual interest that is compounded by increasing vaginal dryness (that rivals the "Sahara-like" vaginal dryness experienced when breast feeding) due to falling estrogen levels. She recommends that perimenopause is "definitely the time to invest in a large tube of safe vaginal lubricant!"

Our bodies also undergo numerous changes around the time of perimenopause, some of which can be triggers for midlife eating disorders. There is a redistribution of body fat to the midsection, gravity takes its toll on many body parts, and it becomes harder to reap the benefits of exercise—with longer hours and more intensity required to keep weight under control. In addition, muscle mass continues to decrease at an alarming rate, and unless weight-bearing exercises are done regularly, many women report feeling frustrated by reduced muscle tone and strength. For women who have suffered from eating disorders in the past, these changes can be enormously challenging and triggering.

Excessive exercise is another avenue into disordered eating in midlife. Women who had developed a certain familiarity with what it took to keep their body in the shape they wanted may suddenly find that that level of energy expenditure is not enough to maintain the shape or size they were accustomed to. They increase their exercise duration, frequency, or intensity in an attempt to maintain their desired figure but then slip into a pattern of excessive exercise that spirals out of control. Injuries that keep them away from exercise create a sense of desperation, which they then counter with either caloric restriction or other unhealthy compensatory methods, such as purging, diet pills, or diuretics. Before they know it, they are in the throes of a full-blown eating disorder.

Other women find that they experience increased or more unpredictable food cravings or urges to binge during perimenopause. Women who may have been able to predict at what time of the month their urges for chocolate were going to increase with their regular cycles have now lost their craving compass as their hormones take on a wacky, often unpredictable schedule. Broadsided by unexpected cravings, they may develop a pattern of binge eating that progresses to BED or even bulimia. This hormonal roller coaster can have the same unpredictable effect on mood. Waxing and waning depression can prompt either unhealthy restriction or binge eating—yet another perimenopausal trigger for disordered eating.

Manopause. Biologically this doesn't really exist, but men go through their own changes as they "cross the border around age fifty." The psychological side is often parodied by the bald man in the hot red convertible, but men also deal with chang-ing bodies and changing metabolisms. Men's weight shifts to the love handles and the midsection; hair thins, disappears, or migrates to parts of the body where it never used to grow; and men too have to work harder to stay in shape. Taking longer to recover after exercise or injury can further hamper their at-tempts to stay in shape. Sex drive can decrease as testosterone wanes, and urges to recapture youth can propel many of the thoughts and behaviors associated with traditional eating dis-orders or the muscle dysmorphic presentations discussed in Chapter 4.

Death of a Loved One. Whether expected or not, the death of a loved one in midlife can touch off eating disorders. Bereavement is a close cousin of depression, and many people find that they simply cannot eat while they are grieving. Some say it feels almost disrespectful or trivial to eat when facing one of the most devastating emotions that we as humans can feel. For some, the loss can be so deeply felt as to question one's own value. Thoughts like "It's not worth looking after myself if he/she is no longer with me" can lead to self-neglect. In extreme cases, not eating can be fueled by an unconscious, or even con-scious, desire to join the loved one in the afterlife: Starvation becomes passive suicide. In most instances, what may look like an eating disorder in this situation stems from bereavement and depression. Although bereavement often follows a natural course, with the pain becoming muted as years pass, it can also intensify and morph into a major depression that requires psychotherapy or medication.

Trauma and Abuse. A difficult topic, but one that cannot be overlooked, is trauma. A substantial minority of women with eating disorders of all types report histories of childhood physical or sexual abuse. This does not mean that abuse causes eating disorders. In fact, the rates of reported abuse are about the same in those suffering from eating disorders as in other major mental disorders. Generally, abuse is considered to be a nonspecific risk factor: It can unleash whatever underlying genetic predispositions to mental illness one may have. But how can childhood abuse continue to be a trigger for eating disorders in midlife? Several possible scenarios exist. Some people experience ongoing memories of the abuse throughout their life. These traumatic memories can be reignited by the smallest of reminders, and the emotions connected to them can trigger disordered eating. For others, the memories and feelings can reemerge when the abuser ages, becomes infirm, or dies— especially if the abuser is a family member. There are certain expectations about the feelings one should have when a family member is passing, but the hurt, pain, and anger from past abuse can dominate at these times. Another common pattern is when past abusive scripts get replayed in the here and now. Being in an abusive adult relationship is mental and physical torture, which is only compounded when it unleashes memories and emotions from past abuse. All of these patterns can trigger predispositions or kindle an eating disorder.

AWARENESS AND ACTION

What are the ingredients of your risk soup? Create your own recipe by constructing a grid of genetic risk factors, genetic protective factors, environmental risk factors, and environmental protective factors and populate it with information about your own life. For example, if you have a family member with an eating disorder (or a suspected eating disorder), depression, or alcoholism, those things would go into the risk genes quadrant. If you have a vigorous metabolism or lots of baseline energy, those would be genetic protection. The environmental quadrants might be more self-explanatory. Risk factors may be some of those mentioned in this chapter, such as loss or trauma, or factors that are unique to you. Protective factors may be a supportive partner, a close community or place of worship, good friends, or living in an area with access to fresh local food—or anything that is health-promoting in your environment. Then, take a close look at your grid and ask which of the parameters are changeable. As mentioned, there's not much we can do about our genes, but we have a better chance of being able to balance out the negative and positive environmental factors. Lastly, develop a plan for change, starting with the most feasible and most likely to be successful target, and give it a try.

PART TWO

Unique Challenges of Eating Disorders in Midlife

CHAPTER 7

Partners Suffer

Before they started living together, Elaine told Eric that she had suffered from bulimia when she was younger, but that she was completely recovered. He had no reason to disbelieve her, but he felt horrible about the fact that she still disliked her body—sometimes intensely—and often required reassurance that her clothes didn't make her look fat. One day when she was at work, he was looking for a book that he wanted to read and checked the drawer of her nightstand. He was shocked when he found it stuffed with a veritable mountain of discarded food wrappers and containers. Everything from cookie wrappers to chips bags to crushed cereal boxes—the drawer was chock-full of evidence that she clearly was not well. Not knowing how to deal with his discovery, he just gathered up all of the wrappers and put them on the kitchen table with a note that said, "What gives?" Then he went to work. When Elaine came home, she was irate and called him on the phone screaming that he had invaded her privacy and had no right to look in her drawer.

Fast-forward to two years after Elaine underwent outpatient individual treatment for bulimia nervosa, and Eric was beginning to think that things were looking up for her health and for their relationship. Although she rarely discussed what was going on in therapy, he hadn't found any more evidence of her binge eating or purging, so he assumed things were going better.

Eric participated in a few sessions with Elaine to discuss how to manage bulimia in the relationship, but he didn't feel like he was part of the process. It was clearly "her therapy" and he was just being informed.

As they were preparing for a reunion with their extended family, Eric noticed that Elaine started asking more often about whether her clothes made her look fat. She was trying on and rejecting lots of outfits and seemed almost inconsolable when it came to trying on bathing suits. Two nights before they left, Elaine asked him to grab her keys out of her purse and he found a half-used package of laxatives. Once again he showed her the evidence and asked how she could betray him and lie to him about her bulimia. He insisted they enter therapy as a couple if they were to have any hope of salvaging their relationship. In their first session, Eric opened with his concerns and asked the therapist, "If she can lie to me so easily about this, what else might she be lying about? Our whole relationship is built on lies."

Relationships in Eating Disorders
As illustrated by Eric and Elaine, eating disorders don't happen in a vacuum; they exist within a social context. Despite stereotypes that women with eating disorders stay single, the data are clear that women and men with all types of eating disorders engage in committed relationships. Some enter into relationships already suffering from their disorder, while others develop an eating disorder after committing. Eating disorders affect relationships, and relationships affect eating disorders. Partners are often at a loss as to how best to help: They feel as if they are walking on eggshells and fear making matters worse. There is no blueprint guiding how to react when their loved one self-starves, purges, binge-eats, or exercises to the point of injury. They don't know what to say when food disappears from the pantry, when their partner skips a meal or goes

to the bathroom to vomit immediately after eating, when they walk in on their wife binge eating after midnight—or what to tell the children, the neighbors, the parents, and the in-laws.

Family meals disintegrate and holidays become nightmares. Partners take over shopping and cooking to reduce the patient's anxiety, and they may gain weight as they attempt to get the patient to eat with them. Their health fails secondary to taking a complete caretaker role, and they hesitate to share the depths of the financial toll the illness takes for fear of exacerbating the illness. The burden on the caregiver is even higher in eating disorders, especially anorexia nervosa, than in other major psychiatric illnesses such as schizophrenia.

One of the pitfalls of lumping anorexia nervosa, bulimia nervosa, and BED together under the general umbrella of eating disorders is that stereotypes associated with one disorder (which themselves are often wrong) get automatically generalized to the other disorders. Nowhere is this as true as in the realm of relationships. For decades, two stereotypes permeated the popular understanding of anorexia nervosa. The first one was that women with anorexia nervosa didn't enter into intimate relationships. The second was that all men with anorexia nervosa were gay. People generalized these erroneous beliefs to the other eating disorders as well, thinking that regardless of the disorder, these were all basically living alone or with their parents, unengaged in romantic relationships. To set the record straight, women and men with all types of eating disorders engage in interpersonal relationships. Moreover, eating disorders don't care if you are straight or gay.

Data back up these facts. We looked carefully at 1,030 women with anorexia nervosa to capture the percentage who were married, separated, divorced, widowed, or living together. Across the following age groups, these were the percentages in relationships, separated, or divorced: (age eighteen to thirty) 25 percent, (age thirty-one to forty) 70 percent, (age forty-one to fifty) 80 percent, and (age fifty-one to sixty years) 80 percent. The same story held when looking at bulimia nervosa and EDNOS.[1] Although the numbers varied slightly, they basically paralleled women in the general population who did not have eating disorders.

A 2012 study of more than forty-five thousand men and women who participated in a health risk assessment shed the first light on relationships in men with binge eating (occurring at least once per month). For men, 77.4 percent of those who reported binge eating and 78.7 percent of those without binge eating reported being married or in a partnered relationship. For women, the figures were also indistinguishable, with 65.6 percent of women who binge ate and 67.2 percent of women who did not binge eat reporting being in a partnered or marital relationship. There were absolutely no discernible differences between men and women with eating disorders and the rest of the population.[2]

Homosexuality and Eating Disorders

Sexual orientation is yet another interesting piece in the midlife eating disorders puzzle. Many of the ideas discussed in Chapter 1 about sociocultural influence on the development of eating disorders have been extended to studies in the lesbian, gay, and bisexual (LGB) population. Such theories suggest that gay and bisexual men may be subject to the same pressures as heterosexual women in trying to sexually attract men and may be more likely to experience body dissatisfaction because community norms place heightened focus on physical appearance. At the same time, lesbian and bisexual women may have lower levels of body dissatisfaction than their heterosexual counterparts and be less susceptible to eating disorders, particularly because they are less influenced by Western ideals for female beauty.

A community-based study in New York City investigating the prevalence of eating disorders in racially and ethnically diverse LGB adults found that gay and bisexual men had a higher lifetime prevalence of bulimia nervosa and other eating disorders than heterosexual men, while there were no statistically significant differences in the prevalence of any eating disorders among heterosexual, lesbian, and bisexual women. They estimated the lifetime prevalence of any eating disorder (anorexia nervosa, bulimia nervosa, BED) to be 8.8 percent among gay and bisexual men and 7.2 percent among lesbian and bisexual women, compared to 1.5 percent and 4.8 percent among heterosexual men and women, respectively.[3] What we don't know about eating disorders in LGB adults could fill libraries.

Quality of Relationships in Individuals with
Eating Disorders
Clearly people with eating disorders are in relationships, but how are those relationships faring? From what we have learned, it's not easy sharing a partner with an eating disorder. Relationship difficulties and distress are common when one member of the couple has an eating disorder. Perhaps unexpectedly, women with eating disorders who are in relationships report more severe disordered eating (e.g., longer illnesses, more attempts at treatments, and more vomiting episodes), as well as more general distress than women with eating disorders who are not in relationships.[4] They also report that they are less satisfied with their relationships and feel less close to their partners than healthy women.[5] Interestingly, body dissatisfaction and marital dissatisfaction tend to go hand in hand.[6]

But are relationships of people with eating disorders any worse off than those of the general population, or than relationships in which one partner has another psychological disorder? Comparing women with binge eating disorder to women with other disorders (such as depression or anxiety), as well as to otherwise healthy control women with no psychiatric disorders, revealed that the women with BED reported lower marital satisfaction and more negative interactions with their partners than the other groups.[7] So it isn't just a nonspecific effect: Eating disorders, in this case BED, seem to be especially challenging for relationships.

We still haven't resolved the chicken-or-egg question here. On the one hand, poor marital satisfaction could be a consequence of the eating disorder. People with BED may isolate themselves from their partners secondary to the shame associated with binge eating, and secrecy, shame, and withdrawal can increase the likelihood of marital conflict. On the other hand, poor relationship quality could increase the risk of developing BED. Binges can be triggered by depression, anxiety, and interpersonal conflict, all of which can then increase the likelihood of binge eating as a means of regulating negative emotions associated with a troubled relationship.

In terms of what comes first, our clinical observations suggest that things shake down in thirds. About one third of couples indicate that the eating disorder pre-dated the relationship, another third indicate that they both started around the same time, and the final third contend that the eating disorder emerged after the relationship. What's particularly relevant is the perception of the partner or the spouse. When a partner discovers that an eating disorder existed before the relationship, and he or she didn't know about it, several emotions emerge. One is a sense of betrayal and lack of trust (as experienced by Eric). Partners wonder why the patient didn't reveal that they were suffering or had suffered from an eating disorder before they committed to each other. The partners may also wonder whether they had been insensitive and perhaps missed major clues that, in retrospect, clearly indicated that the patient was in trouble. Most of the time, when the patient is a woman, the partners basically say they didn't really have a clue as to what was normal for women, when the line into unhealthy was crossed, or what constitutes crossing the line. Jarrod, who discovered his wife had purging disorder three years into their marriage, reflected, "I just thought all women were weird about food. I had three sisters and they were always complaining that they were too fat—even though they weren't—or that they couldn't possibly eat this or that. So I just thought the stuff she was talking about was more of the same. Until I walked in on her vomiting in the shower—then it hit me that we were in the big leagues."

When an eating disorder emerges around the same time a relationship starts, or after the relationship is in full swing, other thoughts can arise. Roberto, whose wife developed serious BED, gained thirty-five pounds, and developed Type 2 diabetes two years into their marriage, racked his brain to figure out what he had done to cause this turn of events. He recalled, "We were really happy when we were dating and even through the first year of our marriage. Then, right after Christmas, things started to change . . . almost overnight. She became withdrawn, spent nights in the kitchen after I went to bed, and cried almost daily about her weight and her health. I just kept wondering what I had done to make her so unhappy. I tried everything, but I didn't seem to be able to do anything to comfort her."

These stories emphasize to us how critically important it is to involve partners, both to help them understand eating disorders and to empower them to be allies during recovery. One of the first things we studied was communication patterns in these couples.

Communication in Couples with Eating Disorders

Communication can become mangled in couples in which one member has an eating disorder. Partners will often say that the eating disorder is the "elephant in the room." While both partners know it's there, the topic is so sensitive, and they are unsure how to discuss it in a way that doesn't do more harm than good. Thus, it often just gets ignored, setting the stage perfectly for an exacerbation of symptoms and delay in seeking proper care.

Couple research reveals that communication is the most

consistent predictor of long-term relationship functioning.[8] A small study showed that patients with eating disorders and their partners engaged in more negative nonverbal communication than did non-distressed couples (e.g., turning away from each other, rolling eyes) and displayed fewer constructive communication skills (e.g., reflecting back what they heard, facilitating the flow of conversation, not interrupting).[9]

In interviews we conducted with couples in which one member had anorexia nervosa, partners discussed feeling caught in a catch-22—as if they were unable to express concern and at the same time unable to express support. They talked about how games and rituals emerged in order to "navigate the traps laid by anorexia." One man recalled that, whenever he made a supportive statement about his fiancée's trying to eat, she heard, "I'm getting too fat, I'm a glutton, and I'm eating too much food." One patient described a complex Ping-Pong game that was played out when her boyfriend was trying to get her to eat. "He'd say, 'Do you want me to fix you something for lunch?' even though I haven't eaten lunch in like nine months. If I said, 'I don't really feel like eating right now,' he'd try to game me and say, 'Well, I'm not going to eat now either.' Then I really can't not eat because I don't want him to go without lunch. It's insane." Her partner explained, "I have to be very strategic all the time . . . like walking through a minefield."

A classic illustration of a phrase that just about every man on the planet has grappled with is a female patient who revealed, "Sometimes I'll say, 'Oh, I'm too fat.' When I say that, I *wish* he would say, 'You're drop-dead gorgeous.' But instead, he gets all practical and says something like, 'You've got to be realistic; you've had three kids.'" This degree of indirect miscommunication and mind reading makes the minefield even more treacherous.

Weight is often the biggest "no-go zone" in terms of communication between partners dealing with an eating disorder, sometimes leading to a complete shutdown of the topic. In a couple in which one member had BED, though both partners were struggling with weight stabilization, every time the "W" word came up, it was met with a stern "This is neither the time nor the place." This automatic shutdown kept the couple from ever discussing how they were going to unite in their attempts to develop a healthier lifestyle.

Eating disorders can be isolating and lonely, yet developing good couple communication is essential to working together toward recovery.

Sex

Healthy sexual functioning is central to the quality of most relationships, but for individuals with eating disorders, it can become deeply entwined with core features of the disorder, such as distorted body image, body dissatisfaction, and shame.[10] Affection, intimacy, and sexuality vary considerably across couples in which one member has an eating disorder. For some, the impact of the eating disorder on body esteem is so pervasive that even basic physical affection is impaired. An action as seemingly innocuous as holding hands or cuddling on the sofa can launch a cascade of negative body thoughts and fear that embracing a simple expression of affection might intensify to intolerable intimacy. For others, affection may be preserved, but sexuality is negatively affected.

Starting with anorexia nervosa, more than 80 percent of patients report difficulties in their sexual relationship.[11] In part, this is related to the fact that anorexia nervosa is often associated with menstrual irregularity, which can be associated with decreased sexual desire. About 60 percent of individuals with eating disorders also report experiencing considerable sexual anxiety,[12] though we don't know to what extent this anxiety is related to body image concerns. If we look across all of the eating disorders, around 40 percent report some kind of sexual discord in their relationships.[13]

Another extremely delicate factor that influences sexuality

is that people with eating disorders can project their own self-disgust onto others and assume that their partners find their bodies as distasteful as they find themselves. Often, this conversation occurs entirely within the head of the individual with an eating disorder, and his or her fears don't come close to approximating what their partners are truly thinking or feeling about their bodies. Carmen, a fifty-three-year-old woman with anorexia nervosa whose husband had gained the sixty pounds that she had lost, stated, "I know he is disgusted by my body, and frankly I am disgusted by his fat." Carmen assumed that her husband was disgusted by her fat, but in reality, he revealed through therapy, he was frightened by her emaciation and was afraid he would "break" her if they had sex.

Carmen's comments about her husband's weight raises another dimension that couples rarely discuss—that is, the extent to which someone with an eating disorder judges her or his partner's physique. Lou, who in his own words was "well padded," said of his wife who had bulimia, "When she looks in the mirror, all I hear her say is how much she hates this part of her body or that part of her body, and how she needs to lose weight here or change the shape of some body part. If she's that critical of her own beautiful body, what must she be thinking when she sees me naked?"

Bryan, who had supported his girlfriend for years while she was in treatment for an eating disorder, disclosed in his second couple therapy session, "All this talk about her body image for four years, and no one ever asked me how I feel about my body. This is the first time I have ever had the chance to talk about my insecurities and what I see when I look in the mirror."

Large body size can also be a barrier to intimacy and sexuality and, if not addressed, can drive a wedge between partners. Janet and Jack had both put on almost one hundred pounds since their wedding day and had only recently realized that they both suffered from BED. When discussing intimacy in their relationship, they told the story of a progression that started with having a romantic and affectionate relationship early in their marriage, marked by a fairly active and satisfying sex life. Yet, as they each gained weight, they became increasingly self-conscious about their own bodies. Each of them started shying away from sex, and eventually they cut out cuddling, and even touching. Jack recounted, "Now on Friday nights, she's on her easy chair and I'm on mine, and we watch cooking shows together. The only shared pleasure we have is food. We'll get that gleam in our eye, and instead of what it used to mean—let's head upstairs to the bedroom—it means let's head into the kitchen and break our diet together. Food is our new sex."

Across all eating disorders, sexual concerns can vary depending on the stage of illness, degree of caloric restriction, body esteem of both partners, and status of reproductive functioning. Irregular menstruation occurs in anorexia nervosa but is also common in bulimia nervosa.[14] We know less about menstrual functioning in women with BED. We do know, however, that sexual satisfaction is inversely related to caloric restriction—so the more you diet, the less satisfied you are with sex.[15] In terms of anorexia, the more weight you lose, the lower your enjoyment of sex,[16] though enjoyment and interest do come back with weight gain.[17] But people with any eating disorder—and even people without eating disorders who go on strict diets—may notice a decrease in their libido. This only stands to reason. It makes sense evolutionarily—it is unwise to produce offspring in times of famine—and it makes sense biologically, as dieting has a direct negative effect on reproductive hormones. That is most definitely not to say that dieting is in any way a contraceptive. In fact, pregnancy can occur even if a woman is not having her periods (see Chapter 8).

Intimacy and sexuality are often overlooked in the treatment of all eating disorders. In part, this must be related to discomfort with the topic or even certain stereotypes held by practitioners (e.g., that people with anorexia nervosa don't have sex or that large people can't navigate sex). Many therapists are not skilled, trained, or comfortable discussing sexuality with their clients, which perpetuates keeping the topic in the shadows. When one is seeing clients individually, it is so important to remember that, outside of the fifty minutes per week in therapy, they face the same challenges as everyone else with regard to relationships. Therapists may need to address their own thoughts and prejudices about sexuality and weight before they can be effective with patients. Addressing affection, intimacy, and sexuality in the treatment of adults with eating disorders highlights not only an important component of relationship functioning but also core features of the eating disorder—namely, body image concerns—within the context of an intimate relationship.

Caregiving

"I've tried everything on the planet, and no matter what I do, I'm screwed," exclaimed Mark when given the opportunity to discuss his role as caregiver for his wife of twenty-five years, who has alternately battled anorexia and bulimia nervosa. Mark vividly illustrates what partners go through as love and compassion are tested by frustration and a pervasive sense of ineffectiveness. As Mark did, partners usually experiment with being gentle or firm, remaining silent or being vocal, and often get to the point of sacrificing their own health for the well-being of the partner.

Most of what we know about caregiving and eating disorders is from research on the parents of youth with anorexia and bulimia nervosa; unfortunately, we know much less about partners and much less about other eating disorders. Studies suggests that individuals caring for someone with anorexia nervosa report greater burden than individuals caring for a relative with bulimia nervosa,[18] as well as poorer general health and greater caregiving challenges than those caring for people with schizophrenia.[19] Most often, caregivers discuss a sense of "loss" of the person they knew and loved before the transformation brought on by the eating disorder. Other topics raised by caregivers include how dominant food becomes in the relationship, the negative impact of the eating disorder on the family, how overwhelming tasks associated with caregiving can become (e.g., in addition to wage earning, having to take over all grocery shopping, cooking, and meal preparation), the loss of a social life, and the impact of the eating disorder on their own health.

Just as parents often report distress, guilt, and helplessness at simply not knowing what to do,[20] partners report similar feelings, coupled with additional domains such as the impact on children and social functioning.

"For the past seven years, it seems our relationship has been about nothing but food," reported Alice, whose husband developed severe anorexia nervosa and obsessive-compulsive disorder after a bout with a severe flu. She described a regimented existence that began every weekend with extensive shopping lists and menu planning that considered both the number of servings her husband needed to get in, plus the high-risk foods he was not yet ready to go near.

In talking about his relationship with his wife, Steve shared, "Every conversation we have somehow manages to come back to food. She won't eat it, but all she ever does is talk about it. We have recipe books and food magazines everywhere, she cooks and bakes for other people, and ironically, she even volunteers in the soup kitchen, but I can't bring her to put a spoon to her mouth. Other people don't have to think and talk about food all the time. I find myself envying men who eat three times a day and even get to go out to restaurants without triggering a major nervous breakdown."

YOU BITE; I BITE

We are deeply social animals. As such, what and how we eat are strongly influenced by our dining companions. People eat more with others than alone, and they match their eating patterns to the people around them. "You take a bite, I take a bite," seems to be more important than even internal sensations of hunger and fullness in determining how much we eat at a given meal.

But what drives this behavior, and does it go awry in people with eating disorders? One explanation is simply imitation or modeling, which is technically called "behavioral mimicry." We do this in many ways, such as mirroring each other's body posture and facial expressions when engaged in conversation. We are hard-wired to copy the actions and mannerisms of others through what's been deemed the "perception-behavior expressway"—that is, seeing an action triggers an automatic response for the very same action. Watching someone frown can lead you to furrowing your own brow, or hearing someone laugh uncontrollably can make you laugh even though you missed the joke. Young adults have been shown to not only take a sip of alcohol directly after their companion, but also to mimic the sipping behavior of actors while watching a movie! This pathway lies at the root of our ability to empathize with others. So why should eating be any different?

Dr. Roel C. J. Hermans and his colleagues at Radboud University Nijmegen in the Netherlands studied whether these same principles applied to eating with a companion.[21] They built a campus laboratory outfitted like a bar and observed the eating behavior of seventy pairs of female college students during twenty-minute meals. One of the participants (the "co-eater") was a plant, and she ate according to instructions to eat a certain amount of food from a preset portion size. Neither she nor the other participant was aware of the ultimate aim of the experiment, though. Not surprisingly, the total amount of food consumed by the members of each pair was very similar. Fascinatingly, however, both women were more likely to take "mimicked bites," or a bite within a five-second interval of the other person's bite, than non-mimicked bites. This pattern held regardless of how much was eaten, the BMI of the participants, or which person was doing the mimicking.

One thing the study could not answer was what was driving this aping. Could it be just another example of the "perceptual-behavioral expressway," or could social comparison be involved? We know that women especially are prone to comparing how much they eat to others around them, to calibrate how much they are eating to socially acceptable amounts. But shared meals are also a fundamental form of social glue: Eating together builds rapport and solidifies relationships. Interestingly, in this study, mimicked bites were three times more likely in the first half of the meal than the second, which could lend support to the rapport-building hypothesis, or could suggest that, as you become fuller, the social mimicry becomes less important than feelings of fullness in determining your eating tempo.

How is this behavioral mimicry interrupted in eating disorders? People with eating disorders are hypervigilant to what others around them are eating and will often strive to ensure that they are eating less than anyone else present. For those with anorexia nervosa, this persists even after the social interaction, while for those with bulimia and BED, this can be followed by a indulgent rebound when they are later alone. Partners of individuals with anorexia nervosa will often gain weight in their attempts to get their loved ones to eat. By trying to "eat with," they may be unconsciously attempting to engage behavioral mimicry. But their loved ones may not be co-eating according to the same principles as healthy individuals, so their attempts to take "a bite for a bite" fall flat—and they gain weight while their loved ones continue to resist the natural tendency for communal eating. Understanding more about how this system is disrupted in eating disorders may help us develop novel ways to incorporate social support into the treatment of those disorders.

Roles and Duty Changes. Jacob described how he had gradually taken over more and more responsibilities as it became clear to him how anxiety-provoking many things were to his wife, Renee. Before she became ill, they had a fair division of labor between them (or so he said; but she often complained that he did less work around the house than she did). After developing BED at age thirty-two, Renee gradually stopped cooking dinner for the family. She found that by buying prepackaged meals and just microwaving them, she could avoid the predinner binges that often took place during meal preparation. Renee recalls, "There were times when I would binge while cooking dinner to the point where there was no food left to serve, and I'd have to go to the store to buy some prepackaged meals anyhow—so I figured, why not just buy them in the first place?" Worried about the nutritional content of overprocessed foods, Jacob began doing a weekly shopping trip on Saturday and planning meals that he would cook for the family. The next wave of problems developed when he would go to cook these planned meals and find that the food he had purchased on Saturday was gone. Renee got home earlier than he did and often found herself bingeing on Jacob's ingredients. As much as she wanted to run to the store to replace the food and cover her tracks, she was fearful of the binge cues she would encounter there. Jacob then changed his approach and shopped on the way home from work, and only for the ingredients he would need that night. This pushed dinner to seven thirty P.M., which he worried was too late for their young boys, but he could find no viable alternative. His kitchen duties then further expanded to making lunches for the boys and basically anything else that involved food. Adding these duties to a forty-five-hour workweek left him completely exhausted and wishing they could go back to sharing household responsibilities.

Health of the Partner. Jacob's full-time job plus household cooking duties left him with very little time for anything else. He continued to maintain outside commitments and was responsible for paying the bills and driving the boys to activities. Any free time seemed to be spent in therapy appointments or, on bad weekends, trips to the emergency room. He was unable to remember the last time he had exercised. Jacob had always been a regular breakfast eater, but his morning responsibilities reduced him to a PowerBar in the car. He'd put on forty pounds and knew he was out of shape when he was out of breath after the uphill walk from the parking lot to his office. His physician was also concerned about an increasing trend in his blood pressure; his father had had a heart attack at forty-eight, and Jacob feared he was heading in the same direction.

Many partners place their own health in jeopardy in an effort to help or support the patients. Much like Jacob, they place their own personal health needs on the back burner due to the urgency and unpredictability of the eating disorder. The most common pattern we have seen in partners of individuals with anorexia nervosa is their own weight gain. They will often "eat with" the patient in hope that having company will encourage their partner to eat. Unfortunately, they're still eating long after the patient has stopped or has purged up the contents of the shared meal. On the other side of the equation, time for exercise gets eaten up by caregiving demands, or partners feel guilty if they are engaging in an activity that is triggering for the patient. If excessive exercise is a trap for their partner, they feel that, by going out for a run, they are "rubbing it in" and being unfair to the patient who has to abstain or restrict exercise.

Sacrifice. After five years of his partner's eating disorder, Josh woke up one day with the stark realization that they basically no longer had a relationship. "We live together, we sleep in the same bed, but life has become putting one foot in front of the other and just trying to survive another day." His partner had gone from being a flourishing advertising executive to, in Josh's words, "a zombie." Matt had been "jolly" when they first met but had been encouraged to go on a diet by a health care professional. Josh had never had weight concerns, but he supported Matt in his weight loss efforts—until he became concerned because the weight kept coming off. Matt's running and cycling got out of control and, when a broken femur led to a bone-density test that revealed that Matt had developed severe osteoporosis, Josh realized he had lost the man he loved to anorexia nervosa. Their social life was nonexistent, Matt was on disability pay, and they rarely shared a laugh and never a meal. Josh compared their life to the lives of friends who had suffered and died from AIDS, except he felt as if he could no longer even communicate with Matt.

Jenny recalled how much her eating disorder had interfered with her and her husband's life as a couple. "The number of times we were planning on going out—to dinner, to a movie, to a birthday party, to a play, even New Year's Eve parties—and I just sat there bawling on my bed, surrounded by clothes, hating how I looked in everything and hating myself. He would just shake his head like, 'Here we go again,' go downstairs, get the remote and sit down in front of the TV. My eating disorder robbed him of a life for a decade."

Self-Care

It is simply impossible to care for someone with an eating disorder without caring for yourself. Desperation is a common feeling when a caregiver realizes that a loved one needs treatment. The initial boost of energy to support the patient in treatment can become strained with the realization that recovery can be protracted and is definitely not linear: Repeated sequences of setbacks, slips, and frank relapses can shake the resolve of even the most loving partner and family. Will recalls, "We went into this thinking she'll get over it, she'll go into the hospital for a few weeks, she'll get out, and we'll move on." If it weren't for a patient therapist who took time to explain the complex course of recovery that is typical for eating disorders, Will might have lost hope during times when his wife's recovery seemed elusive.

Although it was clear to Will that his wife needed support, he was never one to ask for support himself. He tended to be someone who solved problems on his own and shouldered as much responsibility as possible. He figured that the determination that had brought him so far in life would carry him through this as well. Will had little realization, however, of just how uncharted this territory was, and it called upon him in ways that the hardest things he had ever faced—even the death of his own mother—had not approximated. He was overwhelmed with the complexity of treatment (which included dealing with a psychiatrist, psychologist, dietitian, and cardiologist), the frustrating calls with the insurance company, and the emotional roller coaster of family sessions with the social worker. When he agreed to attend a family support session, he felt an enormous relief when he heard other partners sharing their exhaustion, frustration, and love. What Will was unprepared for, though, was the talk about self-care. He was convinced that he needed to spend every waking hour doing something to further his wife's recovery. He had completely missed the fact that taking care of himself was part of taking care of her. He finally started to understand that taking time to do things that helped him manage his fear, stress, and anxiety was directly helpful to the recovery process. He took time to exercise, talked with other partners and parents, and allowed himself some "time off" in order to be more effective when he was with his wife.

Another valuable benefit Will reaped from sharing with other caregivers was how to deal with his sense of shame surrounding his wife's eating disorder. Although he had never quite articulated it, since she developed the disorder after they were married, he feared that other people would point to the marriage as the cause. He was ashamed to admit to other people, and even to family members, that his wife had anorexia nervosa. In fact, he just told them she was in the hospital but never shared why. Being with others in the same situation allowed him to realize that he hadn't caused the disorder, but that he was critical to her recovery.

CARING IS CARING

In 2012, a collaborative project among the University of North Carolina Center of Excellence for Eating Disorders, the Duke Center for Eating Disorders, and the UNC School of Journalism and Mass Communication was developed to encourage parents of children with eating disorders to care for themselves in order to care for their child, but the information is equally applicable for spouses and partners caring for someone with a midlife eating disorder.

The goal of Caring Is Caring is to provide caregivers with the tools to care for themselves during the long recovery process so that they can better support their loved one's recovery. The project's website, www.CaringIsCaring.org, offers resources that clinicians and caregivers have found helpful, as well as examples of self-care activities. The program underscores that caregivers do a lot to help their loved one recover, which, over time, takes a toll on stress levels and physical health, and encourages them to do nice things for themselves, not only to prevent burnout, but to show their loved one that we all deserve to be cared for. It also includes permission and encouragement from the treatment team to engage in self-care, which many caregivers claim was the critical step in keeping them from feeling guilty about "doing something for themselves." Caring Is Caring is based on the belief that self-care helps caregivers feel more confident, supported, and energized, which ultimately enhances their ability to participate in their loved one's recovery.

Here are seven reasons, adapted from Caring Is Caring, why self-care is critical for caregivers:

Reason 1: You will be better able to care for and help your loved one recover.

Reason 2: It is recommended by other caregivers going through the same thing.

Reason 3: It is recommended by clinicians specializing in eating disorders.

Reason 4: It can show patients how to manage their recovery.

Reason 5: You will be setting a good example as a role model for your family.

Reason 6: You will lessen your feelings of helplessness and anxiety.

Reason 7: You can create opportunities to be supported by people who care about you.

AWARENESS AND ACTION

The "Hawthorne effect" refers to a behavior's being improved or changed just by virtue of knowing that you are being measured or studied. For example, we all seem to hit the brakes when we see a police car, even if we aren't speeding. The problem with paying attention to the social aspects of your eating behaviors is that, the minute you start paying attention to it, it will change a little—though not entirely. So whether you have challenges with eating, know or are related to someone with disordered eating, or are just an interested observer, next time you are eating with other people, pay attention to their patterns of eating. Do you see evidence of behavioral mimicry? Does someone at the table seem to be the "pack leader" or the "alpha eater," after whom other people pattern their bites? Is someone, or are you, resisting the flow and actively inhibiting the natural social mimicry process? Understanding how you and others respond to this social hardwiring can help you understand how these forces may influence your eating behavior or the eating behavior of someone you care about.

CHAPTER 8

Pregnancy, Childbirth, and Eating Disorders

Miriam and Gabe had been trying to conceive for six years with no success. After one pregnancy resulted in a miscarriage, they were weighing their options since they both desperately wanted children. At thirty-nine, Miriam was feeling the pressure of her biological clock, but what Gabe didn't know was that Miriam was also quietly terrified of gaining weight during pregnancy. In fact, she worried that the miscarriage had been caused by purging during those early months. Since she had been suffering from morning sickness already, Miriam had rationalized that her body wouldn't know the difference between morning sickness and making herself sick. Her weight was low, but not alarmingly so; Gabe and her obstetrician just thought she was naturally on the thin side. After undergoing a thorough evaluation, they decided to begin fertility treatment including hormone shots for Miriam. The shots made her bloated and nauseated and, probably from years of self-inducing vomiting, she seemed to vomit spontaneously whenever she felt the slightest bit nauseated—which was basically all the time.

Ultimately, they decided to invest the time, money, and emotional energy in a round of in-vitro fertilization (IVF). The physician they were working with was the first one through all of these years of trying to conceive who actually asked Miriam about eating disorders. The doctor noted her somewhat low BMI and gently inquired if she had ever suffered from anorexia or bulimia nervosa. Miriam completely broke down in the office, as the guilt she had been carrying around about contributing to her own infertility came out in her tears. The doctor encouraged her to talk with Gabe and to get treatment for her eating disorder prior to starting IVF. Wisely, she did not recommend spending the time and money on IVF until Miriam's weight and eating were under control. While Gabe had been harboring concerns that Miriam was not fully recovered, the eating disorder had always been "don't ask, don't tell" territory for them as a couple.

Miriam got treatment and found a supportive psychologist (who also included Gabe in sessions, as appropriate) and a dietitian to help her on her recovery journey. After a year, she felt ready to revisit the possibility of IVF, with the support of Gabe, her doctor, and her treatment team. After two rounds, Miriam had a successful embryo transfer and her support system helped her manage the ups and downs every step of the way.

Eating Disorders and Fertility
Human fertility is the end point of a number of complex biological and psychological systems, many of which are disrupted by eating disorders. Energy metabolism, body weight, nutritional state, and reproductive physiology all converge and interact to influence human fertility—in both women and men. Although it is entirely sensible, few people appreciate that appetite and reproductive hormones act in a delicate balance. From a survival perspective, adequate nutrition is important for conception and to ensure robust sperm production. Eating disorders can interrupt fertility in several ways.

The Impact of Eating Disorders on Menstruation. As discussed in Chapter 2, in the old DSM-IV system, amenorrhea, defined as the absence of menstruation for at least three consecutive cycles, was a diagnostic criterion for anorexia nervosa. Extensive research has culminated in the abolition of this criterion in DSM-5, in part because it is so difficult to identify amenorrhea today with so many different contraceptive options, many of which eliminate menstruation entirely; because amenorrhea never applied to men or postmenopausal women; and because copious research revealed that individuals with all of the symptoms of anorexia except amenorrhea did not differ in any meaningful way from women who did experience it.[1]

Even though it is no longer a diagnostic criterion, amenorrhea and oligomenorrhea (irregular menstruation) are common in anorexia nervosa, as well as in bulimia nervosa and BED—despite the fact that these disorders typically occur in individuals who are normal weight or overweight. Clearly, more than just BMI influences menstrual irregularity in eating disorders. Disruptions to otherwise regular menstruation are loud signals that something is biologically amiss.

There are several ways to approach the question of infertility in women with eating disorders. One is to determine the percentage of women seeking fertility treatment who have or have had eating disorders. Although a worthwhile approach, it is complicated by the fact that women with eating disorders may be hesitant to reveal this to a clinician or researcher if their partner is unaware of the eating disorder, or for fear that their provider may delay or withhold fertility treatment. With this caveat in mind, two studies have revealed that between 16 and 20 percent of women seeking fertility treatment have eating disorders, which is markedly higher than the prevalence of eating disorders in the general population.[2]

Another measure of infertility is the length of time it takes to get pregnant while engaging in unprotected sex. The typical window for conception in women in the reproductive years is about three to six months, and a fairly standard definition of infertility is the inability to conceive after twelve months of trying. In a study of 14,663 women in the United Kingdom, women with histories of anorexia or bulimia nervosa were more likely to have sought fertility treatment than women with no histories of eating disorders.[3] But bear in mind that the only women in this study were women who had already become pregnant, so any women who had tried unsuccessfully would not be accounted for. Another study of women with bulimia nervosa indicated that, although many experienced irregular menstruation, it did not appear to affect their later ability to conceive.[4]

Only one study has provided some insight into whether BED is associated with infertility. A group in Siena, Italy, compared eighty-one couples recruited from an infertility center before fertility treatment to seventy fertile controls recruited from an obstetrics and gynecology clinic to determine whether any psychiatric disorders were associated with infertility. Second only to mild forms of anxiety and depression, BED was significantly more common in the infertile group—especially in women whose infertility had no clear biological cause and in women whose infertility was related to polycystic ovaries. The researchers speculate that polycystic ovaries might be related to binge eating and the development of insulin resistance but emphasize that their results are preliminary and that larger studies are required to verify their findings.[5]

The Influence of BMI on Fertility. A very relevant question to address when talking about fertility and eating disorders is to what extent differences in fertility are simply due to extremes of body weight and not a direct effect of an eating disorder. We know from population-based studies that fertility is lower on either end of the BMI spectrum: Both low body weight and high body weight influence reproductive success.[6] Although there are many ways to characterize body size, the measurement that seems to be the most correlated with fertility is the waist-to-hip ratio (WHR). As the WHR increases in women, so does the likelihood of irregular menstruation, and a WHR of 0.8 or greater in women is associated with central fat distribution (or an "apple shape"), which is associated with decreased fertility.

How does obesity affect human fertility? One factor is the balance between androgens (male sex hormones) and estrogen (female sex hormone). Fat itself is a very active organ. Many people think of fat as an inanimate object, but in actuality, in metabolic and hormonal terms it is an extremely active tissue. Fat produces androgens, increased levels of which can interfere with release of eggs from the ovaries, thereby decreasing fertility.

Another family of hormones in delicate balance with reproductive hormones are the appetite hormones. Insulin, ghrelin, and leptin all play a role in both appetite and reproduction. Insulin is produced in the pancreas and plays a major role in metabolizing carbohydrates and fats. Ghrelin is produced in the gut and is an appetite stimulator. It plays a role in initiating meals. Leptin is a fascinating hormone with far-reaching effects on appetite and metabolism. Its primary function is to inhibit eating—to say "that's enough" to the system so that you put down your knife and fork and declare yourself full. Fat cells produce leptin so, logically, people with anorexia nervosa, who are at low body weight and low body fat, have low leptin levels, while people who are overweight tend to have high leptin levels. You can also become "leptin resistant," which means that your body stops being able to "read" and respond to the signals that leptin sends out. All three of these states—low leptin, high leptin, and leptin resistance—are associated with infertility.[7]

But **Eating Disorders Are Not Effective Contraceptives.** Just because a woman isn't menstruating regularly does not mean she isn't ovulating! Many women assume since they are not menstruating regularly that they are not at risk for becoming pregnant. They may shun birth control pills for fear of weight gain, or skip contraception altogether thinking that not menstruating is sufficient protection. One patient, when asked about contraception, stated, "I don't use contraception because I haven't been getting my periods. So I thought I just couldn't get pregnant." Stop the presses! This is completely untrue. We looked more closely at this issue when we noticed, in a large population study, that women with anorexia nervosa were younger at the time of delivery than other moms.[8] This was diametrically opposed to the popular myth that women with anorexia nervosa don't have babies; in fact, in this study, they were having babies earlier. So, we dug into the data and found that a significantly greater number of mothers with anorexia nervosa reported that their pregnancies were unplanned than mothers without eating disorders (50 percent versus 19 percent)—which accounted for the younger age. Since this was a completely unexpected finding, we had not included a question in the original study about whether the women had been using contraception at the time, but it is entirely feasible that they were under the false impression that their eating disorder protected them against pregnancy. In a second large study, almost 42 percent of the women with anorexia nervosa reported having an unplanned pregnancy compared to 28 percent of the mothers without eating disorders.[9] Once again, this suggests that these women might have thought they were infertile.

Anorexia nervosa is not the only eating disorder that is associated with unplanned pregnancies. Women with bulimia nervosa have also been shown in a separate study to have elevated rates of unplanned pregnancies.[10]

This is a worry for several reasons. First, pregnancy prevention isn't the only reason to use contraception. We know next to nothing about whether rates of sexually transmitted diseases are more common in women with eating disorders, although, clinically, we have reason to be concerned. Recently, a colleague who specializes in drug and alcohol counseling with HIV-positive clients reported, "In the last week, we have had two patients, both of whom had a history of bulimia and alcoholism, both of whom had irregular menstruation and didn't use contraception because they thought they couldn't get pregnant. Now both of them are HIV-positive and dealing with an eating disorder." Second, for women with regular menstrual cycles, the absence of menstruation is typically the first concrete sign that they may be pregnant. This (hopefully) triggers a number of behavioral changes, such as stopping smoking and drinking alcohol, taking folic acid supplements, and eating a healthy diet. A woman who is already not menstruating, or is menstruating irregularly, does not have this early dependable warning sign to let her know there's a baby on board. This may delay the point at which a woman becomes aware that she is pregnant, which can also delay these critical behavioral changes, as well as her chance of receiving the important nutritional and emotional support she needs to manage the physical and psychological demands of pregnancy and motherhood.

Pregnancy: The Ultimate Out-of-Body Experience
Julia recounts of her only pregnancy, "Since the age of twelve, when I first developed anorexia nervosa, I had controlled every morsel that went into my mouth and closely monitored every pound my body gained and lost. Even though I was declared 'recovered,' I still weighed myself every day, and if I was up a pound, I regulated my intake to stay in my comfort zone. I really thought that I was ready to have a baby, but when I got pregnant, it was like all the laws of physics and nutrition stopped making sense. I felt like my body started holding on to calories in a different way, and all of my checks and balances went right out the window. I tried hard to remind myself that I was pregnant and had to nourish the baby, but I never really got to the point where I was comfortable nourishing myself and not just eating because of someone else. The baby did fine— she clearly took what she needed to grow—but it was a tumultuous ride for me, and I don't think I can do it again."

As often occurs in medical practices around the world, Chloe's ob-gyn recommended that she go on a diet to lose some weight before becoming pregnant. Her doctor was not aware that she suffered from BED and that this advice was bound to backfire. Chloe's pre-pregnancy diets failed her just as every other diet she had undertaken in the past had. Not wanting to challenge her biological clock any longer, she became pregnant, and her appetite and weight ballooned out of control. She recounted, "I had a fantasy that pregnancy would be a miracle cure for BED—that I would stop bingeing altogether because I was pregnant. But the opposite happened; my binge eating got even worse. I worried about what all of that food was doing to the baby, but then I binged because I was so worried—was my baby going to be fat? Was she going to have diabetes? I had no idea what the consequences could be, so I just assumed the worst, which made me feel even more out of control. When I was diagnosed with preeclampsia, my obstetrician basically gave me an 'I told you so' and admonished me about weight gain and how much my risk for birth complications was going up with each pound I gained. The scare tactics didn't work because I was powerless to control my eating. I finally found a BED treatment group that would take me even though I was pregnant, and I managed to get my eating under some control during the last trimester. Don't let anyone ever tell you that pregnancy is a miracle cure for an eating disorder!"

Weight Gain During Pregnancy. What actually happens to weight during pregnancy in women with eating disorders? Charles, the husband of Sharon, who had to undergo several rounds of fertility treatments before conceiving, exclaimed, "There was a lot of science behind her being able to have that baby." Sharon, with a glint of pride in her eye, said that all of the other women were envious because she gained only four pounds during pregnancy. "They were all ballooning up, and you couldn't even tell I was pregnant. But the baby got all he needed—he just sucked everything from me."

In clinical samples of women with eating disorders, this is not an uncommon pattern. Women who are severely ill with anorexia nervosa who become pregnant struggle to achieve adequate weight gain. Even knowing that they are "eating for two" does not always overcome the deep-seated fear of weight gain. Interestingly, in the general population, when we look at women who have anorexia nervosa but are not necessarily seeking treatment, despite the fact that they start at a lower prepregnancy weight than healthy women, they actually gain more weight during pregnancy. For them, adequate weight gain seems to minimize any adverse pregnancy-related outcomes they might otherwise encounter, and also ensures that the baby is getting the nutrients it needs to thrive.

Thoughts and Feelings About Weight Gain During Pregnancy. So much of the research about pregnancy and eating disorders has been about facts—how much weight gained, what kinds of macronutrients consumed, how many adverse outcomes—but there have been far fewer studies about how women with eating disorders, or histories of eating disorders, think and feel about the experience of pregnancy. As both Julia and Chloe mentioned, pregnancy is an out-of-control experience, and whether you have a history of anorexia, bulimia, BED, or another variation on the theme, when weight is out of your control, anxiety follows on its heels.

Some studies in the United States and United Kingdom suggested that shape and weight concerns decreased during pregnancy in women with active eating disorders.[11] But this is only part of the picture. When you ask otherwise healthy women how worried they are about pregnancy-related weight gain, only 38 percent of them say they are "somewhat" or "very" worried about weight gain, and these tend to be women who are larger going into the pregnancy. Contrast that number with the 89 percent of pregnant women with anorexia nervosa, 91 percent of pregnant women with bulimia nervosa, 92 percent of pregnant women with purging disorder, and 71 percent of pregnant women with BED who are worried about weight gain. These are not subtle differences. Women with eating disorders are worried about weight gain even early on in their pregnancy, highlighting yet again the importance of appropriate support to help them reduce their fears and develop healthy and comfortable eating and weight-gain patterns during pregnancy.

When women with bulimia nervosa were interviewed about their experience during pregnancy, they consistently expressed fears that their child would be affected by their disordered eating, yet this fear did not suffice to prevent ongoing binge eating or compensatory behaviors.[12] They reported varying levels of depression and anxiety throughout their pregnancies, which manifested in fear of uncontrollable weight gain and inability to properly care for their child.

Interviews with pregnant women with anorexia nervosa revealed a range of benefits and consequences associated with the experience.[13] They said pregnancy gave them a sense of normalcy. But most women initially panicked as their weight started to increase and they found themselves suffering from irritability, depression, and anxiety about their weight-gain patterns, even fearing their bodies would not return to their anorexic baseline after pregnancy. While their eating habits did improve somewhat, as they embraced and indulged their hunger with more regular meals and consumed previously shunned foods, these changes were completely attributed to supporting the baby, with one woman commenting, "I'm not doing it for myself, you understand, but have to do it so that the baby will be okay."

Nutrition During Pregnancy. The importance of dietary counseling during pregnancy for women with active eating disorders and histories of eating disorders is crystal clear. During pregnancy, healthy women are encouraged to eat an additional 340 calories per day starting in the second trimester and 452 calories per day in the third trimester to meet the demands of the pregnancy state.[14] The requirements for many micronutrients are increased as well, including iron, folate, and vitamin C.[15] Given the erratic dietary patterns of women with eating disorders, there is concern that they may be unable to meet these greater nutritional requirements.

We'll break the discussion of nutrition down into three overlapping parts—macronutrients, micronutrients, and dietary supplements—in order to paint a preliminary picture of how the diet of women with various eating disorders differs during pregnancy. Macronutrients refer to the basic building blocks of our diet: carbohydrates, proteins, and fats. Micronutrients are vitamins, minerals, or trace elements that are essential in minute amounts for the proper growth and metabolism of a living organism. Supplements are things added to the diet to complement regular intake and can be used to compensate for a deficiency of micronutrients in the regular diet; we'll discuss these separately from micronutrients consumed as part of the diet.

* *Macronutrients.* We know very little about the nutritional status of women with anorexia nervosa, bulimia nervosa, purging disorder, and EDNOS at conception, during pregnancy, and in the postpartum period. Some studies suggest that intake for women with anorexia nervosa during pregnancy may include less protein and fat than healthy women.[16]

We have somewhat more information about women with BED, primarily because the disorder is more common. Women with BED reported eating more total energy (calories), total fat, monounsaturated fat, and saturated fat during pregnancy than healthy women without eating disorders. They also reported lower intakes of juice and fruit but higher intakes of candy, fats, and milk desserts than women without eating disorders. This is of some concern because high consumption of sweets early in pregnancy is associated with excessive gestational weight gain,[17] as women with both bulimia nervosa and BED are at risk for excessive weight gain during pregnancy.[18] The effect of these dietary patterns is not limited to the mothers: Babies born to women with BED are also at greater risk of being large, and their mothers are at increased risk of needing to deliver by cesarean section.[19]

* *Micronutrients.* Of the micronutrients, folate has probably received the most press, due to its critical importance in protecting against neural tube defects. However, other micronutrients such as iron, B vitamins, vitamin A, and iodine have also been linked to pregnancy outcomes and fetal neural development. Even more important may be the extent to which a woman is deficient across multiple micronutrients.[20] We do not have sufficiently large studies of women with anorexia, bulimia, and purging disorder to draw definitive conclusions about micronutrient status, but we can surmise that if these eating disorders remain active immediately before and during pregnancy, vital micronutrient stores may be depleted. In our large study in Norway, published in 2011, we were able to document that women with BED had a significantly lower intake of folate, potassium, and vitamin C than healthy women.[21]

* *Supplements.* Supplementation may serve a critically important role in pregnancy for women with eating disorders whose diet may be deficient in some of these fundamentally important micronutrients. In this same Norwegian study, we found heartening evidence that women with eating disorders are taking supplements at some point during their pregnancy. With the standard among healthy women being 95.5 percent, the following percentages of women with various eating disorders reported some supplementation: anorexia (91.2 percent), bulimia (92.2 percent), purging disorder (93.2 percent),

and BED (90.6 percent).[22] Although there's still room for improvement (even among healthy women), at least over 90 percent of all women were supplementing their diet with essential micronutrients during pregnancy.

The problem comes when we look back to the fact that pregnancies among some of these women are unplanned, and they may not realize they actually are pregnant until well into the first trimester. Since supplementation during the first trimester is so critically important, many healthy women will commence supplementation when they are trying to become pregnant so that they have all the necessary micronutrients on board before conceiving. When we look at supplementation rates in the two months before pregnancy, the numbers are more concerning. Whereas 44.3 percent of healthy women report supplementing in that interval, the numbers for women with some eating disorders are also lower: anorexia nervosa (38.2 percent), bulimia nervosa (43.9 percent), purging disorder (30.2 percent), and BED (38.3 percent). So the real focus for improvement should be in those months preceding conception, and presumably in the first trimester as well.

What Happens to Eating Disorder Behaviors During Pregnancy?

How does pregnancy affect eating disorder symptoms? The news is neither all good nor all bad. Early optimistic reports offered hope that pregnancy seemed to provide at least temporary relief from eating disorder symptoms for most women. This relief was short-lived, however, as women report that symptoms return after delivery.[23] Anecdotal reports tell us that, much like smoking or alcohol use, many women find themselves able to abstain from their disordered eating behaviors for the duration of the pregnancy. For some, they find they can hold the symptoms at bay "for the sake of the baby," but after the birth, when the baby is no longer inside, they are often unable to sustain the change. As is true with all behavior change, when undertaken because of an external, temporary reason, it is unlikely to endure. But not all women are able to control their disordered eating behaviors during pregnancy, and for the ones who can, it is not always an easy road.

Three large studies that have looked carefully at eating behavior during pregnancy in women with eating disorders have provided us with a richer picture of what happens to eating disorders symptoms during this period. In the large Norwegian study, which included women with BED, bulimia nervosa, and purging disorder, between 29 percent and 78 percent of women reported remission of their eating disorder during pregnancy.

About one third of women struggling with eating disorders believe that pregnancy could provide a means to recover from their disorder,[24] even though they are aware that the pregnancy-related weight gain will feel out of their control. They also state that weight gain and a larger body size are more acceptable during pregnancy than under other circumstances.[25] Unfortunately, the belief that pregnancy will somehow launch their recovery is not well founded.

Several studies report that women who have *recovered* from eating disorders experience relapses during pregnancy. So, rather than a window for remission, pregnancy served as a window for relapse. A Swedish study of women with anorexia nervosa prior to pregnancy found that 33 percent experienced a sufficiently severe relapse during pregnancy to warrant contact with a psychologist or psychiatrist.[26] Likewise, a study in the United Kingdom reported that women with past eating disorders reported an *increase* in overall concerns about weight and shape during pregnancy.[27]

Even more worrisome is the fact that pregnancy seems to be a risk period for the onset of BED in women who did not have the disorder before becoming pregnant. Although the exact reasons are unknown, the risk was highest in women who had low social support, had lower incomes, and whose native language was not that of the country in which they lived.[28]

There appears to be some awareness that behaviors such as self-induced vomiting and laxative abuse may be harmful to the pregnancy. Women with anorexia nervosa tend to report low rates of these behaviors in pregnancy, but higher rates of excessive exercise to control weight (defined as greater than one hour of moderate to vigorous activity daily) than reported by healthy women during pregnancy.[29] Women with bulimia nervosa have also been shown to substitute one compensatory behavior for another along the same lines (i.e., trade in laxative use for excessive exercise).[30]

Nausea and Vomiting. Another very logical question is to what extent women with an eating disorder marked by self-induced vomiting are likely to develop nausea and vomiting during pregnancy. That is, if someone is vomiting frequently because they have bulimia, are they more likely to be susceptible to nausea and vomiting during pregnancy? Hyperemesis gravidarum is a condition marked by extreme, persistent nausea and vomiting during pregnancy that may lead to dehydration. Women with purging-type eating disorders may be at increased risk of hyperemesis and they are significantly more likely to report both pregnancy-related nausea and pregnancy-related vomiting than women without an eating disorder.[31] Women with these problems should be closely monitored to ensure that the severity of the symptoms does not lead to inadequate weight gain and nutrition.

Birth Outcomes in Women with Eating Disorders:
The Impact of the Eating Disorder On the Baby
If women with anorexia nervosa who come from general population samples (i.e., they are not identified by the fact that they are in treatment) are able to conceive and gain adequate weight during pregnancy, they do not appear to have increased complications with most aspects of delivery. There are no increases

in preterm births, gestational hypertension/preeclampsia, induced labor, vacuum extraction, use of forceps, or breech presentation in women with past or recent anorexia nervosa. Some studies suggested that they had a higher rate of cesarean sections, while other studies did not. Women with more severe, active symptoms of anorexia nervosa during pregnancy may be viewed as high-risk by their obstetricians, resulting in more frequent cesarean sections. Earlier case studies of treatment-seeking women with severe anorexia nervosa throughout pregnancy reported significantly worse outcomes on all measures (including intrauterine growth restriction, preterm delivery, small for gestational age, high occurrence of breech presentation, increased vaginal bleeding, and low Apgar scores).[32]

Women with both recent and past anorexia nervosa do give birth to babies with lower birth weights than healthy women with no history of eating disorders,[33] which is not surprising given that low birth weight is associated with lower pre-pregnancy BMI. Yet while birth weight may be significantly lower, no differences have been found in Apgar scores at five minutes for babies of women with anorexia nervosa compared to babies of healthy women. Sufficient weight gain during pregnancy seems to play a crucial role in preventing starvation-related adverse birth outcomes.

In our large Norwegian study, mothers with anorexia nervosa reported greater weight gain than mothers without eating disorders, suggesting that, in light of their lower BMI before pregnancy, they were gaining appropriate amounts of weight during their pregnancy.[34] Potentially due to this adequate weight gain, we did not see evidence of worse birth outcomes for women with anorexia nervosa compared with a healthy referent group. Thus, in clinical practice, monitoring of gestational weight gain throughout pregnancy in women with past or present anorexia nervosa appears to be critical and may mitigate against adverse outcomes.

Information on birth outcomes of women with bulimia is

mixed. Some population-based studies have shown little increased risk, whereas clinical studies have shown higher rates of miscarriages and lower birth weights.[35] Mothers with BED, in contrast, have babies with higher average birth weight, have a higher risk of their babies being large for gestational age, and have a higher risk of cesarean section births than healthy control mothers; but most of the effect seems to be due to higher pre-pregnancy BMI rather than to BED itself.

The Postpartum Period
The transition to motherhood is accompanied by dramatic physical and environmental changes. The following section will discuss issues related to eating disorders during the postpartum period, including postpartum dieting and body image, perinatal mental health, and breast-feeding.

Postpartum Dieting and Body Image. Caring for a newborn baby can be stressful, and sleeping and eating can be seriously affected, even in women without eating disorders. New mothers are also often home alone, which can increase the risk of engaging in previous disordered eating behaviors—especially when the mother is sleep-deprived and stressed.[36] Western culture has created another bubble of discontent around postpartum weight loss. Nearly half of new mothers report dissatisfaction with their weight during the postpartum period,[37] and the increased body fat and loss of abdominal muscles from pregnancy can reignite dissatisfaction with body shape and weight. At nine months postpartum, women who report body dissatisfaction are more likely to report overeating or poor appetite, worse mental health, and bottle feeding (vs. breast-feeding).[38]

Women with anorexia nervosa and purging disorder lose weight more quickly during the postpartum period, which either reflects a fundamental difference in their biology or suggests that they may be resorting to restriction, compensatory measures, or other extreme weight-control behaviors to get back to their pre-pregnancy weights. The majority of women who do experience relapse after their baby's birth attribute their return to disordered eating to the desire to lose weight and to feeling fat. Without the motivation to eat "for the baby," women with anorexia nervosa may find it difficult to continue to eat for their own health. In contrast, women with BED appear to hold on to their pregnancy weight longer after birth.[39]

Postpartum Depression and Relapse. We have already discussed the fact that all eating disorders commonly co-occur with depression and anxiety disorders. For all women, the postpartum period is a high-risk time for depression. Distinct from the "baby blues," which can manifest as mood swings, crying spells, anxiety, loss of appetite, and trouble sleeping and are experienced by upward of 80 percent of women, postpartum depression is longer-lasting and more severe and may include any of the aforementioned symptoms, as well as lack of interest in the baby, thoughts of hurting oneself, or thoughts of hurting the baby.[40] It is estimated to occur in one to four pregnancies out of one thousand in the general female population. But women with anorexia nervosa are at greater risk, with 36.1 percent experiencing depression during their pregnancy and 45.5 percent during the postpartum period.[41] These rates are comparable to women who suffer from major depression who do not have eating disorders. Furthermore, women with a history of anorexia nervosa are over-represented in clinical samples of women seeking treatment for postpartum depression.

There is room for optimism. About a third of women who had eating disorders during pregnancy report being in remission at eighteen and thirty-six months postpartum. Thus pregnancy can launch recovery for some women. The other two thirds either continue to experience lingering symptoms or experience a full-blown eating disorder. These numbers suggest that the postpartum period might be an important pivot point for intervention. Reaching women during this malleable phase may allow us to boost the percentage of women who remit rather than continue to experience disordered eating.

TRAUMA AND ABUSE HISTORY

Women with eating disorders, especially the binge-purge type, are more likely to report histories of trauma and abuse than women without eating disorders.[42] Trauma and abuse histories also independently increase the risk of depression during and after pregnancy, as well as other psychiatric disorders. The combination of a history of abuse and an eating disorder seems to be a particularly strong risk combination for postpartum depression.[43] Thus, special care should be taken to educate women with comorbid eating disorders and trauma history about the increased risk for postpartum depression and pregnancy complications, and proactive mental health care is especially critical for these women.

Breast-feeding

From the very first days, mothers with histories of eating disorders will worry that if they are unable to feed themselves properly, they will never be able to trust themselves to adequately nourish their children. Doubts can creep in even at the earliest stage when mothers are deciding to breast- or bottle-feed. Women with eating disorders tend to be less likely to breast-feed and then tend to discontinue breast-feeding earlier than women without eating disorders.[44] Although the precise reasons for this are unknown, our clinical experience provides some cues.

There are myriad reasons why women with eating disorders may choose not to breast-feed. Women with anorexia nervosa, bulimia nervosa, purging disorder, and other eating disorders often have concerns that they will not be able to produce enough breast milk. In part, this is because of their fears about what the eating disorder may have done to their bodies, but more often, it is related to whether they believe they will be able to consume adequate calories to maintain breast-feeding. Moreover, if a woman is strongly driven to return to her pre-pregnancy weight, it may be more important to her to get to the gym and go back on a diet than to struggle with the uncertainties of breast-feeding. A third reason is that breast-feeding is an amazingly intimate experience between mother and child. For a woman who has deeply ingrained body dissatisfaction or even body loathing, this frequent intimate contact may simply be too overwhelming and distressing. Some mothers with eating disorders also contend that they are not prepared to sacrifice their bodies for breast-feeding; they cannot tolerate the possibility of the wear and tear that the breasts endure during breast-feeding and the long-term consequences on appearance. Finally, some women have reported considerable anxiety about not knowing how much milk their children are getting if they breast-feed. Not being able to see or measure an actual amount fuels their concerns about underfeeding or overfeeding their children. For these mothers, bottle-feeding and schedule feeding seem to be the preferred method. For some who really want to breast-feed but have this concern, pumping and measuring can be an option, although this requires spending twice as much time to first pump and then feed with a bottle, often making it unsustainable.

As is so often the case, lactation consultants are rarely schooled on eating disorders, and mothers are hesitant to bring this up in the hospital or at follow-up visits. Further education of lactation consultants about the impact of eating disorders could assist with developing support mechanisms to help women through some of their anxieties and give them the opportunity to breast-feed if they so chose. Difficulties with breast-feeding may also be due to the increased risk for postpartum depression and anxiety in women with anorexia nervosa.

Reproductive Counseling for Women with Eating Disorders
This section first reiterates the reasons reproductive counseling is needed for women with eating disorders, and then provides the health care provider with helpful tips on how to have "the conversation" with a patient. It can also be useful for the patient to help guide how she raises the topic with her physician.

As reported earlier, women with anorexia nervosa do become pregnant and are more likely to have unplanned pregnancies. The take-home message for providers and patients is that absent or irregular menstruation does not preclude pregnancy. Therefore, special attention should be paid at routine ob-gyn visits to inform patients with eating disorders about the possibility of pregnancy, even when at low body weight, in order to ensure that they are making informed decisions about their reproductive health and that they understand their need for family planning.

Providers should discuss the use of contraceptives and vitamin supplementation with women with eating disorders of reproductive age. Although oral contraceptives are often prescribed in order to restore menses and prevent bone loss in women with anorexia nervosa, data do not support this clinical practice to protect against osteoporosis.[45] Their use can also obscure our ability to determine the natural weight at which menses return. However, in addition to preventing sexually transmitted diseases, the use of barrier contraceptives (i.e., condoms) may prevent unplanned pregnancy in sexually active women. Furthermore, given the fact that women with anorexia nervosa who experience unplanned pregnancies are likely nutritionally depleted at conception, routine visits should include counseling about the need for daily vitamin supplements and adequate fat and protein intake to ensure optimal absorption of micronutrients.

Reproductive counseling is also needed in cases of infertility. Of patients who present for treatment to an infertility clinic with absent or irregular menstruation, 58 percent met clinical indicators for eating disorders, but none had disclosed these problems to their providers.[46] In another clinical sample, 60 percent of infertile women with ovulatory dysfunction had anorexia nervosa, bulimia nervosa, or EDNOS. Therefore, appropriate infertility treatment also includes detection and adequate treatment of an eating disorder. Treating anorexia nervosa first, through proper nutrition and weight restoration, is an important first step in infertility treatment, potentially saving significant costs, stress, and complications associated with assisted reproductive technology. In addition, when patients with active eating disorders pursue infertility treatment, such technologies may also be less effective than in healthy women.

   Having the Conversation. Considering that the first thing that happens at an ob-gyn appointment is that a nurse asks the patient to step on a scale and then records her weight, this is an ideal time for nurses to discreetly raise questions that start discussions about eating disorders. Just watching a woman's response to the scale can provide mountains of information about her feelings about her weight. Asking her questions about how she feels about her weight gain rather than simply presenting guidelines or admonishing her for gaining too little or too much would make the interaction around weight infinitely more therapeutic and informative.

   In a survey of ob-gyns, just over half (54 percent) believed that assessment for eating disorders fell within their scope of practice, but a large majority (88.5 percent) rated their training in assessing eating disorders as barely adequate. However, almost all generalists (90.8 percent) agreed that eating disorders can negatively impact pregnancy outcomes.[47] Unfortunately, most mothers with histories of eating disorders (64 percent) do not reveal this information to their ob-gyns. Of those who did discuss their eating disorder with their provider, only half perceived the discussion to have been beneficial.[48] With knowledge about a patient's history of eating disorder, clinicians can make appropriate accommodations, including reducing appearance-based comments by themselves and their staff and modifying weight assessments to include blind weigh-ins. Most ob-gyns do not know what to do if a patient reveals a history of eating disorder—so they prefer not to ask. The most important course of action is a referral to a therapist and a dietitian experienced with eating disorders.

Mental Health Treatment
Given the increased risk of perinatal depression and anxiety in women with current or past eating disorder, additional screening for symptoms of depression and anxiety is also important, as appropriate treatment for these conditions is critical to the well-being of both the mother and the newborn-to-be. The practice guidelines of the American Psychiatric Association and the American College of Obstetricians and Gynecologists recommend outpatient psychotherapy, such as cognitive behavioral therapy (CBT) or interpersonal psychotherapy (IPT) in cases of mild to moderate depression and anxiety (see also Chapter 11).

However, women who are suffering simultaneously from eating disorders and severe depression and anxiety symptoms may require pharmacological treatment, including antidepressants and anxiolytic medications. There are no specific guidelines for the treatment of women with coexisting eating disorders and depression during pregnancy, but it is recommended that psychiatrists carefully assess maternal-fetal risk and discuss these risks with their patient before initiating psychotropic medication use either during pregnancy or postpartum.[49] However, practice guidelines were developed for women with perinatal depression without consideration of eating disorder status, and we do not yet have data to guide the treatment of depression and anxiety in pregnant women with eating disorders.

In sum, effective care in the ob-gyn setting during the preconception and perinatal period should include: 1) screening, assessment, and documentation of eating disorder history and other comorbid psychiatric history; 2) education about the possibility for pregnancy in the presence of amenorrhea, the need for supplementation, and the increased risk of perinatal depression and anxiety in women with eating disorders; 3) a collaborative discussion of patient emotions and weight assessment options at clinic visits; and 4) referral to a multidisciplinary team of mental health providers and dietitians for treatment, as appropriate.

AWARENESS AND ACTION

The media place unrealistic expectations on women to return to their pre-pregnancy body weights almost immediately postpartum. Tabloid reports of celebrities reaching their prepregnancy weights only two to six weeks after giving birth send the message that you, too, can and should get your old body back that fast. In *The Woman in the Mirror*, I emphasized society's push to erase all traces of pregnancy and motherhood from our bodies. Apply your media watchdog skills to see how the media set up unrealistic expectations. If you are pregnant or postpartum, give yourself a break, allow your body to recalibrate naturally, and focus your attention on your relationship with your child, rather than on a misplaced societal prescription for weight loss.

CHAPTER 9

Parenting with an Eating Disorder

Two weeks after Sasha was born, Melanie felt like she had to get back to running. She recalled that she couldn't stand being cooped up at home with the baby all day and not exercising. Taking walks with the stroller didn't satisfy her intense need to exercise. Her pregnancy weight wasn't coming off as fast as she wanted, and Melanie felt trapped at home. Melanie recalled in tears that Sasha would be crying in her crib, but she wouldn't pick her up until she finished two hundred sit-ups. She bought a jogging stroller so that she could start to run with the baby when she was just one month old. Once she got out on the streets, even though she intended to keep it to a few miles a day, she just couldn't put the brakes on increasing her mileage. When winter set in, she was up to six to ten miles per day, and she just bundled three-month-old Sasha up more. Her husband, Cullen, didn't know she was running with Sasha, but one cold day in February, he was driving from one job site to another and saw them running about five miles from their house. Melanie recalled him pulling the car over, grabbing Sasha, feeling her cold little hands, and accusing Melanie of trying to kill their child. He filed for divorce, claimed Melanie was endangering the life of their child, and ultimately got sole custody of Sasha. The eating disorder robbed Melanie of her marriage and her daughter.

Most adults with eating disorders would give anything to protect their children from developing eating disorders. In all my years of clinical practice, I have never heard a mother or a father who wanted their child to endure the same torture they had. What I have heard, though, are desires for their children to never be teased about their weight (as they had), to not become overweight or obese (which they would have difficulty dealing with), and to not be aware of their own eating disorder. What comes up most often with eating disorder patients are questions about how to buffer their children from risk. Parenting with an eating disorder is not easy, and there are very few research studies to guide parents or clinicians about how best to help. Much of this chapter is rooted in common clinical sense and experience and not necessarily based on scientific literature.

How Can I Feed My Child Properly If I Can't Eat Properly Myself?

One reason why feeding is such a difficult and emotionally laden issue for many parents is because parenting and food are hard to separate. From the minute our children are born, we are programmed to make sure they get enough food. This is the primary role of parenting, especially with young children. As many of you probably know from your own families, most mothers never stop worrying about whether their children are eating the right amount and types of foods.

Parents with eating disorders struggle to differentiate between normal eating phases and a developing eating disorder. We frequently receive calls from mothers who worry that their children's picky eating is the first step down the path to an eating disorder. It's better that they're concerned rather than oblivious, but too much worry and too much vigilance can backfire. Often they may fear that they see behaviors or attitudes in their children that remind them of their own youth or their descent into an eating disorder. Sometimes this might be an accurate perception, but other times it can be overidentification and a complete misinterpretation of what is actually going on with the child developmentally. On the other hand, patients sometimes worry that if they make too big a deal of their children's eating, they might trigger an eating disorder.

Ellyn Satter[1] has advised generations of mothers on feeding their children. She emphasizes that while children are born with some innate eating capabilities, they have to learn others. The trick is to not interfere with those innate skills and to teach the ones they need to learn. Children are born with the drive to eat, the ability to self-regulate based on hunger, appetite, and satisfaction, and the ability to grow in the way nature intended. Most children have an internal sensor for how much to eat, but the actual amount they eat can vary enormously from meal to meal. Parents with eating disorders (and even parents without eating disorders) often focus too narrowly on intake at one specific meal, when the best way to examine your child's eating is from a bird's-eye view. If a child has a big breakfast, she might naturally regulate and have a smaller lunch. While this little lunch might be worrying, if you step back and look at it in terms of a whole week of food, instead of meal by meal, you realize that a very intelligent mechanism is keeping the child's daily intake fairly steady over time. Understanding these natural patterns can help reduce worry about those meals when a child isn't very hungry. His or her body might just be doing that internal math that helps balance overall caloric intake.

One pattern we have observed with mothers with eating disorders is a tendency to give their children "special diets."[2] This can be anything from organic to vegetarian to non-processed. There is nothing inherently wrong with this approach, and in fact there may be distinct health advantages—unless it becomes overly rigid. When parents become hypervigilant to what their children are eating to the point where it interferes with their social lives, this can present a whole new set of problems.

Curtis insisted that the whole family eat only organic and nonprocessed foods. This edict included packing snacks when his son, Jacob, went to parties or friends' homes, and Jacob was never allowed to buy school lunches. When he was younger, Jacob didn't really care all that much, until the other kids started teasing him about being a "granola cruncher" and a "bark eater." Wanting to prove to his friends that he was normal, Jacob started eating junk food just to "show them." Curtis once caught him with Oreo cookies when he arrived to pick him up from a birthday party, and he reprimanded Jacob. The boy was completely trapped between his dad's demands and taunting from his peers. Curtis is probably doing his family a favor by insisting they eat a primarily organic diet, but increasing flexibility and allowing for occasional deviations would save Jacob from teasing, as well as eliminate his desire to rebel. Rigidity is typically driven by anxiety, and it is better to address the underlying anxiety than to just keep tightening the screws.

When strict food rules are driven by children, the picture can become more complicated. A mother recovering from a recurrence of her adolescent anorexia came panicked into a therapy session, frantic that her fifteen-year-old daughter wanted to become a vegetarian. This alarmed her primarily because vegetarianism had been her own first step toward anorexia. She recalled telling her own mother that it was because she was against cruelty to animals, when the truth was that she was petrified of the caloric density of meat. She knew anorexia could be deceptive and worried that her daughter was giving her the same line that she had given her own mother. We worked through the problem, and the mom noted that she had not seen any additional concrete alarm bells. She also reported that her daughter had recently watched the film *Food, Inc.*[3] in biology class, which had started the whole conversation about vegetarian eating. The session ended with the mom realizing that she was indeed still the mom and had the authority to discuss and make decisions with her daughter, rather than just giving in to her desires—which could complicate her own recovery. Together, they ended up negotiating an acceptable outcome, which was to reduce the amount of red meat they ate and increase their consumption of sustainable fish. Mom held fast to not being able to cook two meals for the family every night and reminding her daughter that she will be able to make decisions like this on her own when she is adult, but that because she was only fifteen, this type of decision had ramifications for the whole family. In this case, the daughter was not falling into an anorexic trap and had just been positively influenced by the movie. The final negotiation was a healthy outcome for the whole family.

Restricting is not the only concern. Alec e-mailed me worried about his seven-year-old daughter, Alicia, who had developed a pattern of secret eating. While cleaning her room, he found food wrappers under her bed, and when he looked in their spare freezer in the garage, he found that packs of all sorts of bulk foods (like muffins, cupcakes, and other breakfast foods) they had bought at their wholesale club store were half eaten. Alec called himself an emotional eater, but he had never gone so far as to identify himself as a binge eater; and now he was genuinely worried about Alicia developing similar patterns. He claimed Alicia had never seen him eat for comfort and said they didn't have strict food rules in the house. Most of the foods she was eating in secret fell into their Sesame Street–inspired "sometimes foods" category. In Alicia's case, the family had just moved to a new state, and she was having some challenges making friends in her new school. I encouraged Alec to focus on how she was feeling about school, and at this point not to focus as much on the food—but to keep a watchful eye out to see if the sneaking food abated when the transition became smoother. Although things did settle down, this early experience suggested that eating might be a manner in which Alicia will try to deal with emotional issues, in much the same way her father does. If it emerges again, Alec will not hesitate to get a proper evaluation and intervention to prevent Alicia from developing a lifelong pattern of turning to food in times of stress.

Too Fat, Too Thin, Just Right? How Can I Tell?
Ellie simply could not tell what was normal. How was she supposed to tell if her children were the correct weight when she had never been able to accurately appraise her own body size? The constant comments and advice from relatives and neighbors just made her head spin. Labels like "string bean," "baby fat," "growth spurt," "lanky," "chubby," "cream puff," and "Gumby" had all been used to describe her son and daughter at various stages of development by everyone from grandparents to complete strangers. To most moms, these would be considered nothing more than innocuous albeit stupid comments that people make all the time, but for Ellie, every one of them set her off in an obsessional tailspin.

We simply do not understand the perceptual disturbances behind anorexia nervosa. Both anorexia nervosa and muscle dysmorphia, or "reverse anorexia," are associated with individuals seeing something different in the mirror from what others see when they look at them. Typically, as far as we know, their perceptions of others are not as skewed. Two intriguing studies shed some light on how they perceive others. One study revealed that people with anorexia nervosa show an aversion to fat rather than an attraction to thinness when looking at others.[4] The second study used a clever technique that asked individuals with anorexia nervosa and healthy control participants to judge whether they could fit through an image of a projected doorway on a wall. Although patients with anorexia nervosa were more likely than the controls to judge themselves as being too large to pass through the door (even when they would have easily fit), they had no trouble making these judgments for other people's bodies.[5] Whether this holds for perceptions of their children's bodies remains unknown.

A few studies have suggested that mothers with bulimia nervosa are more likely than healthy mothers to view their daughters as overweight and to encourage them to lose weight.[6] Regardless of whether mothers actually did pressure their daughters to lose weight, the daughters' perceptions of maternal pressure to do so are predictive of eating pathology,[7] but so much more work needs to be done to truly understand these relationships.

Although the data are scarce, I am grateful to several parents with eating disorders who have shared with me details about the inner turmoil they experience when it comes to the physical appearance, shape, and weight of their children. These are not always feelings about which they are proud; in fact, many of them were ashamed as they spoke of their innermost thoughts and feelings.

Perhaps the most difficult topic for mothers with eating disorders to discuss is how their own personal body dissatisfaction can bleed over to their perceptions of their daughters. Amelia realized at one point that she had taken to visually body checking her daughter in much the same way that she physically body checked herself. One day, her daughter came downstairs in low-cut jeans and a cut-off shirt, and Amelia saw that she had developed a "muffin top." She felt horrified that her daughter had gained weight and felt deep pressure from inside to do something about it. Amelia held her tongue, but she overidentified with her daughter to the point that she felt as if it were her own fat. She wanted to go up and grab it and then keep body checking her daughter to see if the muffin was getting bigger or smaller. Instead, Amelia found herself constantly looking at her daughter's middle, visually checking. She didn't know what to do. She wanted to comment on her daughter's weight gain—in fact, she wanted to put her on a diet—but she was well aware of the dangers of going down that path. So all she did was suggest that her daughter not show so much skin because it was against the school dress code. Even when her daughter covered up, though, Alicia was still preoccupied with her daughter's waistline.

Fathers who are hypervigilant about their own body fat can also be challenged by their children's developing bodies. When exercise and minimizing body fat start taking on moral overtones in their minds, fathers can become critical of their children if they don't follow suit and remain fit and lean. At times, the quest for leanness and muscularity can take on a near-religious fervor, and family members who don't get on the exercise bandwagon can be criticized as lazy. Even if words aren't spoken, silent disapproval can be equally as damaging. It can drive kids toward their own pursuit of muscularity, or drive them in the opposite direction, rejecting the rituals and rigidity that govern their parent's life.

For all of these parents, we encourage them to differentiate between their "accepting voice" and their "critical voice." Maybe that internal critical voice focuses on the muffin top or the undesirable layer of body fat, but the expressed accepting voice has to gain an upper hand. The accepting voice is the parent who loves the child for all that he or she is, who focuses on all aspects of the child, rather than just physical appearance, fitness, or thinness. We encourage parents to actively cultivate the accepting voice, with the goal that it become louder than the critical one. Simply squashing or denying the internal critical voice is unlikely to be effective, but bolstering the positives has a higher likelihood of keeping those critical comments from escaping over time.

"They Don't Know . . ."

All the parents with an eating disorder whom I have met have underestimated how aware their children are of their disorder. The belief that you can hide binge eating, restriction, or purging from your children is false. As parents, we spend so much time teaching our children how to follow the rules of the table: eat what's cooked for you, eat everything that's on your plate, finish your vegetables, don't inhale your food, don't play with your food, don't hide your broccoli under your mashed potatoes. As a result, our children are keenly attuned to whether other people are following those same rules. If Mom cooks for the family and then doesn't eat with them, you can be sure that the children notice. Or if Dad eats small portions at dinner and then heads downstairs for a binge later, the kids definitely know that Daddy always has a big snack at night. They are acutely aware, and in fact, they may be more aware than you are. The checklist on page 202 is an inventory of the types of things parents may consciously or unconsciously do that children might notice.

Most parents with eating disorders will ask, "Should I tell my child about my eating disorder [or my history of an eating disorder]?" This has to be a highly individualized decision and depends on many factors. In the best of all non-stigmatizing worlds, it would be as easy to tell a child about an eating disorder as it is to say "Mommy has high blood pressure," or "Daddy has high cholesterol." But that is not our world (yet), and parents are keenly aware of how much children talk and how easily health information can be misunderstood. On the one hand, knowledge is best and knowing that you have a family history of a disorder can be a helpful ingredient in prevention. On the other hand, you can provide too much detail too soon, before children are developmentally capable of understanding. If the disorder clearly interrupts your family life, then the children will have to have some details because their imaginations can conjure something much worse than the reality. By the time they reach adolescence, for many it is valuable to hear about their parents' histories or current problems. What tends not to be effective is putting offspring in the position of "parenting" a parent with an eating disorder. This blurs boundaries and disrupts the chain of parental authority and can interfere with the effectiveness of parenting by someone with an eating disorder. There are many, many individuals with eating disorders who are

Parent Inventory. Which of these behaviors are you concerned about?

Possible Concerns	Yes, I am concerned about this
Only eating a limited variety of food	☐
Body snarking comments (e.g., my thighs are fat)	☐
Not allowing certain foods in the home	☐
Not eating with the family	☐
Eating other foods than the family eats	☐
Enforcing rigid dietary rules for the whole family	☐
Feeling uncomfortable during meals	☐
Can't enjoy meals with your child because you are distracted	☐
Not "all there" during meals (e.g., because of anxieties about food or feeding)	☐
Having trouble telling when your child is hungry or full	☐
Sneaking food for yourself that you don't want your child to eat	☐
Comments about calories/fat/carbs during mealtimes	☐
Body checking behavior (e.g., critiquing self, pinching waist)	☐
Describing foods as good or bad, labeling foods	☐
Excessive exercise	☐
Food rituals	☐
Binge eating in secret	☐
Running to the bathroom to purge after meals	☐
Limiting own foods for your breast-feeding child	☐
Discomfort with child's fluctuating appetite	☐
Worry about additives, preservatives, nonorganic foods	☐
Eating less than the rest of the family	☐
Other behavior:	☐

excellent parents, just as there are many people with diabetes, cancer, asthma, anxiety disorders, and any number of other medical conditions who are exemplary in their parenting role.

"My Child Is Getting Chubby—What Should I Do?"
Without question, the most common challenges faced by parents, both with and without eating disorders, is dealing with an overweight child. Whether your child received a BMI report card from school, is screened as overweight by her or his pediatrician, or gets teased in school about weight, or whether you or she notice that she is overweight, the next steps are not clear. I routinely get calls from fathers asking how they should talk about this with their daughters. They simply do not know how to bring the topic up without stepping on a land mine. Parents have more difficulty talking with their children about weight than about alcohol, drugs, or sex.

What makes parents so reluctant to talk to their children about the risks of being overweight? Many don't think it's a problem until their children are obviously overweight, says family psychologist Susan Bartell, Psy.D., in a WebMD report.[8] "But the next issue I see often is parents are really afraid they will trigger an eating disorder." She adds, "And then the other thing is they don't know how to talk to kids about weight. They think they will hurt their kids' feelings or damage their self-esteem." And kids aren't making this talk any easier. Nearly three fourths of them (72 percent) say the discussion would be more embarrassing to them than to their parents.

We're not afraid that a discussion about sex, drugs, cigarettes, or alcohol will damage our children's self-esteem or trigger some sort of a disorder. In fact, the opposite is true: We think that discussing these topics will foster and preserve self-esteem. Conversations about those topics could actually protect our children from situations that could be deeply damaging to their well-being. Why is weight so different? Neither parents nor their children have a blueprint for how to talk about weight without engaging all of the peripheral topics that make it so electrified, such as self-image, personal responsibility, mood, affect regulation, and stigmatization. It's easy to stand back and say we should just be able to have nonemotional, objective conversations about weight, but we all know that's not going to happen.

We need more data on what conversations to have and how to have them. Opinions we have; data, we have not. We need evidence-informed guidelines about how physicians should discuss weight and BMI with parents, and how parents can discuss these topics with their children. I had a conversation with a pediatrician colleague and friend of mine recently about this topic, and she reminded me that there is no opportunity for a pediatrician to talk with a parent without the child in the room unless the child is an adolescent—so whatever is said about weight is heard by the child. Sometimes, she said, she needs to speak in code with the parent—but we know how attentive little ears are in that situation. Thus, guidelines must address how to have these discussions with younger patients present and with adolescent patients either present or out of the room. A follow-up phone conversation can provide the necessary privacy.

Just the words that we use to discuss weight can have an effect on patients' ability to hear them in a motivating and not a judgmental way. When asked what terms they were uncomfortable hearing from a physician when discussing weight, patients responded with "fat," "excess fat," "large size," "obesity," and "heaviness." Patients found terms such as "weight," "BMI," "weight problem," and "excess weight" to be more palatable.[9]

So, we often tell parents just to focus the conversation on healthful eating and physical activity. There is a lot of merit to that approach, but what if our children want to talk about weight? Do we have an obligation to discover a way to discuss weight without engaging all of those peripheral charged topics that make it such an uncomfortable and embarrassing topic?

The Rudd Center for Food Policy and Obesity (www
.YaleRuddCenter.org) has a rich array of tools to help parents
talk with their children about weight. Some of their key recommendations include: focus on healthy changes in your child's
behaviors (such as eating more fruits and vegetables) and not
just on weight loss; make healthy changes as a family, as they are
more likely to be effective; be aware of labeling language that
further stigmatizes obesity; watch out for making negative comments about your own body size; avoid "should" statements—
such as "you should eat this" or "you should eat that"—and
instead make an alternative recommendation; encourage self-
esteem and remember that it comes from many areas, not just
appearance; identify triggers for your child's eating (e.g., stress,
boredom, anger), talk with him or her about it, and assist with
finding healthier ways to deal with those emotions; and be a
support partner for your child, always celebrating successes, no
matter how small.

There are going to be many individual differences in how
best to approach this topic with children, but that should not
thwart our investigations into how to have a conversation about
weight. Our research agenda should be driven by neither opinion
nor fear, but rather by the overarching need to determine how
best to advise physicians and parents on this important topic.

Eating Disorder or Not, You're Still a Parent
What parents with eating disorders often lose sight of is that,
despite their eating disorder, they are still parents, and with
that comes the right and the responsibility to exert parental
authority. I have seen extremely ill women and men be highly
functional parents. Those are the people who can effectively
ring fence their eating disorder from their identity as parents
and not allow it to infect their parenting identity with self-doubt.
Other parents may be less effective at drawing this distinction
and become concerned that their eating disorder will invariably
render them ineffective at parenting. The truth is that the eating

disorder may affect your parenting. You may be fatigued, have difficulty attending events where food is served, or miss events because of appointments or hospitalizations; and your children may have to deal with their fears about your illness and their inability to completely understand what is wrong with you. All of this aside, you can still be a good parent: You can still teach your children right from wrong, you can still dole out appropriate discipline, you can still give them comfort and love. It is only stigmatization that makes anyone think that someone with an eating disorder cannot be a good parent. I have never heard anyone contend that someone with arthritis can't be a good parent, or that someone with irritable bowel syodrome can't. Why should eating disorders be any different?

Support Team

What you need to be an effective parent with an eating disorder is a strong support team. Your partner needs to work with you as a co-parent, and he or she may need to pick up the slack during particularly troubling times. You need a pediatrician with whom you can discuss your concerns about the impact of your disorder on your children and who can help you to calibrate your own perceptions of them and concerns about their growth and development. You may well need a family therapist to help the entire family deal with the impact of an ill parent on family functioning. You may also need to enlist the help of family and friends during difficult times to assist with child care or driving when you are unable to carry out these tasks.

The Impact of Recovery on Family Dynamics

If a mother or father is suffering from an eating disorder, family systems develop and often calcify around the illness. As you recover and new patterns emerge, families can resist change. It is not uncommon, when the "identified patient" starts to recover, for problems to surface in other family members. Sometimes families are in "crisis mode," and everyone is able to suppress his or her own problems when one member is particularly ill. Once that person shows signs of recovery, however, others can start fraying. Partners may become depressed, children might have more difficulty at school or with peers, and just as you start to get a foothold on your own recovery, you might find yourself having to also take on more of a caretaking role as these new problems emerge. Recovery is not all a happy homecoming. Many feelings have been put on hold, and many sacrifices have been made in service of the eating disorder. Whereas it is not safe for those feelings to come out when you are still ill, as you recover, you may be perceived as sufficiently robust to deal with others' problems. This can be a difficult time for all family members and one in which external support may be especially critical. Eating disorders do take hostages, and sometimes the feelings associated with these changes need to be processed before families can completely heal.

AWARENESS AND ACTION

This little game is called "What Would You Say?" As parents and grandparents we are often caught off guard by questions from our children, comments by others, and even comments by physicians, who, although well meaning, may not be optimally sensitive. Some of the following scenarios have been posed by parents who asked how we would recommend dealing with them. Others are examples prepared by the Strategies to Overcome and Prevent Obesity Alliance (STOP; www.stopobesity alliance.org). First give it a go yourself, and then look at some of our recommendations. Thinking about these situations in advance can provide you with confidence when they actually come to pass. It is important to tailor your answers to suit the age of your child and to make sure the interaction is a real two-way conversation, not a lecture.

Scenario	What Would You Say?
Your child comes home and says, "I'm fat. I want to go on a diet."	
At a pediatrician's visit, routine BMI screening indicates that your child is in the obese range. Your pediatrician says, "You have to put him on a diet."	
Your child comes home crying from school several days in a row and starts refusing to go on the bus. She says that a group of girls have started to tease her about her weight.	
You come from a culture in which the natural body shape and size are larger than the "Western ideal." Your daughter comes home and says she hates not looking like her thin classmates.	
You overhear your son tease another child for being fat.	

Scenario	What Would You Say?
Your daughter wants to stop eating dinner with the family and just take a salad up to her room.	
You notice that your child tends to turn to grazing in the pantry the night before tests.	

Question	Sample Response
Your child comes home and says, "I'm fat. I want to go on a diet."	**In response to "I'm fat," you could:** *Elicit more information:* "Honey, you've never said this before [or you've been saying this more often]. What's been going on that is making you think this way?" *Express values/acceptance/love:* "We are all made to look different, and to have unique attributes on the inside and out—that's what makes us beautiful and interesting. You're great at solving puzzles, listening, and you're energetic and spunky [add special attributes here], which makes you fun to be around—these are the reasons people like you and are drawn to you. Changing your body will not change these things about you that I so love and admire! You are so much more than your body. You're a neat package of all of these things." If the child mentions there is a particular body part he/she is dissatisfied with, you can focus on what that body part has allowed him or her to accomplish: "You were blessed with strong arms that allow you to swim extra fast." or "Your legs are what allow you to run and jump so far." **In response to "I want to go on a diet," you could try:** *Elicit more information:* "What do you mean by 'going on a diet?' Tell me what going on a diet means to you." [Often this is a very fuzzy concept in children's minds and they really don't know what they are saying. Establish a non-diet mentality and challenge the notion that dieting is healthy.] *Express concerns/values/focus on health:* "You know, we just had a checkup with your doctor and she thinks your body is healthy and functioning pretty well. Dieting can really mess up your body. In fact, it doesn't work very well and can be very dangerous. If you are interested in eating healthier we can talk about what that might look like as a family and try out some new

	snacks and family meals together. It's probably good for everyone in our family to think about how we can eat better. What do you think about that plan?"
At a pediatrician's visit, routine BMI screening indicates that your child is in the obese range. Your pediatrician says, "You have to put him on a diet."	**You could try a two part response:** *To your child:* "Honey, what the doctor is saying is that we, as a family, can all work together to come up with some fun ways to make sure we all stay healthy. We could all benefit from moving our bodies some more and eating more healthfully. When I was a kid I took a father-daughter dance class with my dad. Let's brainstorm some creative ideas that we can do as a family to be healthier?" Then you would follow up with the doctor afterward (not in the presence of your child) and inform him or her that the term "diet" is counterproductive and it is preferable to focus on health habits and other physical indicators of health (vitals, labs, etc.), not weight loss as an outcome measure. You could refer your physician to the Academy for Eating Disorders "Guidelines for Childhood Obesity Prevention Programs" at http://www.aedweb.org/AM/Template.cfm?Section=Advocacy&Template=/CM/ContentDisplay.cfm&ContentID=1659.
Your child comes home crying from school several days in a row and starts refusing to go on the bus. She says that a group of girls have started to tease her about her weight.	**You could try:** "Kids like to find whatever they can to tease each other about and it's NOT okay. Those kids teasing you obviously don't know you, but if they did, what do you want them to know about the kind of person you are, the person that I see and the people who love you so?" [Try to elicit some positive self-statements.] *Elicit more information and validate her or his feelings while expressing your values:* "I'm really sorry that happened to you. I can see you are upset and that's understandable. It's absolutely not okay to make fun of other people, especially because of how they look. It makes those kids look really uncool! What do you think about what they said?" Listen for response. "You

	know what IS cool? It's really cool that every one of us is made differently; we are all different shapes and sizes, have different personalities, and are good at different things. I love your big smile, witty sense of humor, and your love of the arts [add specifics here, such as you are really good at choreographing dance, drawing pictures, and making pottery]. You are beautiful just the way you are!"
	You could work toward a mutual solution: "Let's come up with a good plan for how to handle this, okay!?" Then discuss options, including (for your child) not rising to the bait or finding a safe friend to sit with on the bus (and for you) talking with the bus driver, calling the children's parents, talking with the school administration, or all of the above.
You come from a culture in which the natural body shape and size are larger than the "Western ideal." Your daughter comes home and says she hates not looking like her thin classmates.	*Elicit more information:* "Let's talk about what kinds of things are happening that are making you feel that way?" *Express your values:* "You're right, we are different. But everyone is different in some way, whether it is their size, shape, hair color, skin color, personality . . . the world is made up of all different types of people. What you see in the media doesn't accurately portray that: It makes us think we have to all strive to look the same—thin, young, and 'flawless.' The media makes us think there is something wrong with us. But, you know, in our culture, we think beauty comes in all shapes and sizes, and we really value diversity. Unique equals beautiful. Same equals boring. Differences are what make us interesting." You might also refer to family and friends from the same culture whom she admires and open a conversation about all of the ways they are each unique and beautiful.

You overhear your son tease another child for being fat.	*Lay down the law:* "Honey, let's sit down for a sec. How would you feel if someone said that to you? Not so great, right!? It is absolutely not okay to tease people—whether it is about their looks, smarts, athletic ability, etc. We just don't do that. In this house, we are respectful and appreciative of everyone's differences—including differences in how they look. I don't ever want to hear you teasing someone again."
	"You might see other kids tease each other, but you are a lot better than that. Teasing is not okay; it only hurts other people and it will make you feel bad too, because I know you aren't the kind of person who wants to hurt others."
Your daughter wants to stop eating dinner with the family and just take a salad up to her room.	*Elicit more information:* "We always have dinner together, what's more comfortable for you eating by yourself?"
	Express your values: "We rarely get to see each other, and family meals are a time for us to swap stories, plan the weekend, relax, and enjoy trying new foods together. I like to hear about all the amazing things that you are doing. It's my job as a mom/dad to make sure you are getting adequate nourishment and I can't do that if you don't eat with us. So, family rules are actually important for everyone's health and well-being . . . family meals continue!"
	"You need a lot of energy to get work done and be an active kid. A salad isn't a balanced meal and won't give you the energy and nutrition you need to focus and be so active."

You notice that your child tends to turn to grazing in the pantry the night before tests.	*Elicit information/express concern/offer solutions:* "Hey sweetie, I just want to check in. How are you feeling about this test coming up? When I was your age, I would get pretty darn nervous before exams. My heart would race, my shoulders would tense, and I would often worry that I hadn't studied enough or that I would forget everything during the test. Does any of that sound familiar? Do you ever get a little tense or anxious?" ... "I found some ways to help me cope with my anxiety that might help you too" [then discuss options]. "Sometimes when I get stressed or worried, I want to find something to make me feel better right away. Do you think snacking helps you feel better in the moment? Does it help in the long run? Let's talk about how it's working so we can figure out if there might be other ways to help you when you are feeling [insert emotion here]."

PART THREE

Your Journey
to Recovery

CHAPTER 10

Motivators for Recovery

In the remaining chapters, I am going to be speaking directly to people with eating disorders. These chapters emerge from my own clinical experience and decades of working with people with all forms of these disorders. Although addressed to them, the information is also critically important to caregivers and providers so that they can work together with patients to tailor a unique journey to recovery.

Ultimately, recovery is optimal when it is motivated by your own desire to reclaim your life. At its core, recovery has to be for you. Eating disorders represent a particular challenge in this arena, however, largely because of the low self-esteem that is often part of the clinical picture. If you have anorexia nervosa you might believe you don't deserve to eat; or if you have bulimia, you might be ashamed by your purging behavior; or if you have BED, you might think you're disgusting and shameful because of your overindulgence. If so, you may feel unworthy of recovery—as if you deserve the punishment that is an eating disorder for eternity. If you wait for recovery to be for you and only you, it may never come. With a nod to the Beatles, however, "we get by with a little help from our friends"; that is, you can launch and bolster your recovery process by seeking and accepting help from your friends. If we draw on recovery stories around the world, several themes emerge regarding who those friends are. It remains important that recovery be solidified by the belief that you have the right to recover, but for many that is too big for a first step.

How the recovery journey begins varies from person to person. For some, there is a definitive turning point—an event or a moment of inspiration or fear that jolts one out of the eating disorder status quo and onto a path toward health. For others, it is a cumulative effect of a series of smaller events or decisions that ultimately culminates in a new direction. Whichever profile is more accurate to your situation, one steadfast truth is that every recovery journey is unique. Just as no single treatment fits all, no single model for recovery fits all. Your recipe for recovery has to be tailored to you at a specific time in your life. As such, the following sections do not provide a pat "recipe for recovery," but rather present some observations about recovery from midlife eating disorders.

Aikido of Ambivalence
Perhaps with the exception of substance use disorders, eating disorders are unique in that those who suffer from them are often very ambivalent about letting go of their symptoms. Unlike people with anxiety disorders ("Doctor, please take this phobia away") or depression ("Doctor, please help me lift this dark cloud from my head"), people with eating disorders often enter therapy with one foot inside and the other outside the door. They may only partially disclose their symptoms, clinging to one or a few behaviors to allow them to continue managing their anxiety, or controlling their weight, or regulating their mood— whatever function that eating disorder symptom is serving.

I often liken this hesitation to trying to drive a car with one foot on the accelerator and one foot on the brake. One half is ready to embark on the journey, but the other is not ready to relinquish control. Ambivalence is part of the eating disorder, and thus, dealing with ambivalence has to be embraced as part of the recovery process. Direct wrestling with ambivalence is rarely effective, and attacking it directly can often send shards underground, only to resurface later in treatment and further hinder progress.

I prefer an "aikido approach" to ambivalence, both as a provider and as an approach for patients to deal with their own uncertainty. Aikido is a Japanese martial art that has roots in martial studies, philosophy, and religion. By blending with the motion of the attacker and redirecting the force of the attack—rather than opposing it head-on—aikido allows practitioners to defend themselves while simultaneously protecting their attacker from injury. The aikido approach to ambivalence is akin to the "rolling with resistance" characteristic of motivational interviewing (see Chapter 11).

There may be some areas of change that are easier to address at certain points, and some doors that are slower to open. Rather than sending a battering ram through the closed doors, sidestepping them and amassing smaller victories with doors that are wide open or ajar allows you to start developing a library of change that can build momentum for opening the doors that are sealed shut. The part of aikido that is of particular value is protecting the attacker from injury. The point of recovery is not to be bludgeoned into behavior change, but to get there without injury; the first principle of any treatment, after all, is to do no harm. By acknowledging that ambivalence toward recovery serves a protective function and by "rolling with it," you can simultaneously experience change while also maintaining some semblance of familiar security.

Cleaning Your Room
During the recovery journey, it is not uncommon for things to get worse before they get better. Someone with anorexia nervosa might lose weight during the first week of hospitalization. Although this might not satisfy the insurance company, it could be, for example, because she or he was "water loading" (i.e., drinking a lot of fluid to increase weight) at home and basically spent the first week reestablishing fluid equilibrium.

You might come into treatment for bulimia or BED binge-eating twice a week and, two weeks into treatment, as you begin to explore difficult thoughts and feelings, find that your rate of binge eating or purging increases rather than decreases. This is all completely natural. Recovery is rarely linear.

I vividly recall Saturday mornings when my mother would threaten to throw everything on the floor of my room into trash bags to be taken to Goodwill unless I cleaned up my room. I was not the tidiest of adolescents. Having reached the point of no longer being able to stuff anything more into my drawers to disguise my mess, I faced the horror of actually having to clean my room thoroughly. Before I started the reorganization process, I would pull everything out of my drawers, and in the process of tidying, things would first get a heck of a lot messier. I would sit there on the floor, surrounded by piles of clutter and clothes, overwhelmed by the task and wondering how I was ever going bring order to the chaos—and thinking of a million other things I would rather be doing on a Saturday morning. But then, after my period of despair, I would develop a game plan, start sorting things into logical piles, and methodically putting them away, slowly clearing the floor. The end product was a tidy room (plus one junk drawer, which I have always had to keep for those un-categorizable things) and a happy mother.

This metaphor is exactly like the beginning of the recovery journey for many people. Maybe you have settled into some sort of illness equilibrium, where your symptoms are serving some psychological purpose but you have avoided hospitalization. As you start peeling away the layers of your symptoms and uncovering the thoughts and feelings they have been suppressing, eating disorder behaviors might increase—leaving you with that overwhelmed feeling of being surrounded by piles with no exit strategy. This too is natural—uncomfortable, yes, but predictable. You have been trying to heal broken bones with Band-Aids for years. When you finally take them off and realize how much healing there is to be done, it can feel positively overwhelming.

It is at this point, when you are feeling most vulnerable, that you and the people around you need to exhibit the most patience and compassion. Acknowledging being overwhelmed and rolling with this feeling allows you to see how you have gotten to where you are and fully appreciate the depth of the recovery process. Just as with cleaning your room, a quick fix would be to stuff your clothes willy-nilly back into the drawers and slam the drawers shut—but the next time you were looking for your blue sweater, it would be hard to find, buried beneath underwear, and hopelessly wrinkled. The same goes for recovery: You could walk away from treatment and carry on, but the messy symptoms would still be there.

The good news is that, after the overwhelmed phase, you can start to envision how to organize and plot your recovery journey. Taking small steps, taking one day at a time, and tackling aspects of wellness that are most tolerable to you can begin to bring order to chaos and help you regain control. When ambivalence sets in and starts pulling you back to the familiarity of the eating disorder, it is worthwhile to take inventory of reasons you may have to take the first step toward recovery . . . and then keep going. Some of the motivators that many midlife patients have shared are presented below.

Children and Grandchildren
Recall Alita, who stated that when she was seriously ill, she had deluded herself into believing that her anorexia nervosa had no impact on her children? Coming to terms with the fact that her eating disorder was visible to them, that they feared for her life, and that her disorder was wreaking havoc on their childhoods was a strong motivator in her recovery. Even though eating disorders have strong biological bases, in the recovery process, there are choices every step of the way. Alita recalled

the constant battle in the early stages of recovery (and at times later on) when she would be faced with a choice. "Either I lie in bed and succumb to this misery and depression, skip breakfast, and let my husband feed them frozen waffles, or I haul my butt out of bed and force myself to go down there and be with them and eat." Alita got out of bed not because of herself, but because of the thought that her illness was creating childhood memories of Mom's never being there for her children in the morning. This worry propelled her to act in the opposite way of how she was feeling: to go downstairs, face her fears, and be there for her children. As Alita explained, "Every morning, I struggled to 'make it about them' and not about my disorder. Anorexia is a selfish bitch. She ruined my childhood, and I wasn't going to let her completely ruin my children's childhoods, too."

Perhaps the most eloquent campaign for the positive impact of grandchildren on your recovery journey comes from Australian author, advocate, and blogger June Alexander. In a moving blog excerpt, she described what it was like to enter the swimming pool for the first time with her grandchildren, letting go of the decades of self-consciousness that had kept her out of bathers (a swimsuit by any other name!). From June's blog:

> This afternoon, I surprised two of my grandchildren, aged five and two. For the first time, they saw me in a bathing costume. They laughed, and so did I. They laughed a lot more when we entered the indoor swimming pool. The five-year-old had a large water pistol and proceeded to shoot me. The only thing was, he was laughing so much he could not see straight and luckily missed his target much of the time. The two-year-old, resplendent in her pink "Tinkerbelle" bathers, took to the water like the plastic yellow duck and three baby ducks that her mum had given her to play with, and I was busy keeping up. (Mum is expecting baby

number three in three weeks and was looking on from the poolside—she was laughing, too.)

For an hour, we frolicked in the indoor pool like seals in the sea. Happy, happy, happy. Why was this simple event so important to me? Because I let it happen! When my daughter was aged five years, she gallantly swam 50 metres in the "big pool" as a junior member of the local swimming club in the town where we lived. I made sure she and her brothers had lots of opportunities—swimming, ballet, Brownies, Cubs, tennis, horse riding lessons, and more. But I never once got in the pool and played with my daughter or her brothers. Or went to a rehearsal, or went to a gymkhana, or went camping with them. Not once. The rigidity of thought imposed by decades of eating disorders prevented me doing many things that I knew I would have enjoyed, and wanted to do, but could not allow myself to do.

Back to the swimming pool—my grandson was so impressed at having my company in the pool that when I suggested maybe it was not such a good idea to shoot Grandma in the eyes with that water pistol (because I needed to keep an eye on his little sister, proper little fish that she was), he took off his goggles and said, "Here, Grandma, put these on." To be offered goggles by a young grandson is very special indeed. I loved swimming as a child. Growing up by a river in rural Australia, I swam several times a day during the summer holidays—together with the snakes, goannas, platypus, salamanders, bearded dragons, eels, and whatever else had made its home in the river. I love water. Full stop. I love to look at it, hear the sounds (of rain, waves, rapids) and most of all, being in it. If only my grandchildren knew what great medicine they are for me.

MORE WISE WORDS FROM JUNE ALEXANDER ON GRANDCHILDREN AND RECOVERY

I invited June to offer more comments on the role of grandchildren in recovery, and she provided me with these anecdotes that underscore the central role that the third generation can play in crystallizing recovery and keeping guilt from polluting newfound liberation from an eating disorder.

> I spent today "in the past" doing something I have wanted to do for a long time. The time was right to do it. I got out my family photograph albums. Since age eleven, when I got my first Brownie box camera, I have been the creator and keeper of pictorial records in my family. The albums number more than fifty, and there are hundreds of pictures. Today, I leafed through each one, pausing, remembering, and occasionally slipping one out of its cover and placing it in a special pile on my dining table as the first step in creating a book keepsake for each of my four children. The task was easy enough, turning pages. But it was loaded with reminders of my pervasive eating disorder.
>
> I stared in disbelief at pictures of each of my children with their annual birthday cakes. The children looked glum, even when about to blow out their candles. Their countenance was downright solemn. I calculated the years. Yes, I was in my thirties and forties, lost in the dark forest of my eating disorder, trying to find the way out. Counting calories, checking weights. Lost. At home and on family holidays, my illness ran amok. Binge, starve, good day, bad day. Moods seesawing. Reflected in the faces. I felt desperately sad for my children and sad for me. We each missed out on much time with each other. I tried to be a good mum, as best I could with the small amount of "me" not

consumed by the eating disorder, but my illness obviously had affected my children—and their dad. He looked glum, too. Not even saying "Smile for the camera!" could raise a grin from anyone. The pictures told the story.

Oh, hurry, hurry, through the albums to 2006. The year I regained me. Smiles: genuine smiles. My children are adults, becoming parents now; pictures of grandchildren begin to appear. Smiles, h-a-p-p-y and free. No eating disorder clouding, sabotaging relationships. I'm living in the moment (*"Come on, Grandma, it's time to play!"*). I squeeze through the tunnels in the playground and whiz down the toddler's slide, granddaughter squealing with glee on my lap. Throw shells in the waves. Plant carrot seeds in the garden. Blow bubbles, lots of bubbles, and chase them, too. Everyone is smiling. Including me. The pictures tell the story.

How lucky I am, that my children stayed by me, that their dad provided stability and security for them when I was too sick to do so. Today my children are my carers, recovery guides. Their children are the cheer squad.

The children are a strategic part of my maintenance team; they are mini-carers, stress-relievers, hug-a-lots, happiness-givers, non-judges, living-in-the-moment experts. ("Grandma, please help find this Lego part"; "Grandma, you are my favourite when Mummy is at work"; "Grandma, help me with this puzzle—sit on the FLOOR beside me, Grandma!"; "I want you to come and read FIVE stories when I'm in bed tonight, and there is room for you to lie beside me, Grandma.")

Do I have a take-home message to share? Yes. Never give up on recovery.

For more wise words from June's blog, visit www.june alexander.com/blog.

Relationships

Zane got to the point where he just couldn't tolerate the deception anymore, saying, "My eating disorder has robbed me of authenticity in friendships." Having grown up in Northern California, he joked that within three minutes of meeting someone, you start sharing intimate details about your psychotherapy. Although he wasn't looking for a return to that flash intimacy, he was distressed by the fact that his bulimia had brought a dimension of secrecy into every friendship and relationship he had had over the past fifteen years. "There was always a third person in the room, and that was bulimia. I would be out to dinner, supposedly engaged in the conversation, but half of my brain was just trying to time my trip to the bathroom so I wouldn't be caught out. I'd be lying in bed with my girlfriend on Sunday morning only half paying attention to her, focusing on how much I really needed to be out on the bike to keep my body fat down. Every single one of my friends had to share me with my eating disorder. It was selfish, and I got tired of it."

Zane pinpointed the fact that eating disorders occur in a social context. For many, relationships form the cornerstone of recovery and are a strong motivator for wellness. Later in treatment, Zane recalled, "I forgot how intense friendships could be. The bulimia had sort of insulated me from the emotional part of friendships. I almost had to relearn how to be empathic and understanding, and how to accept that from other people. I had been in emotional Bubble Wrap for fifteen years."

Fear

Patti had been hospitalized for purging disorder more times than she could count. Years of laxative and ipecac abuse landed her in the emergency room and medicine wards in multiple cities across the country. She feared there was a "Wanted" poster in every ER in the country with her mug shot on it. During her last admission, she ended up in the ICU with kidney failure, yet her physician's admonition that she had to stop doing this to herself or she was going to die had no effect. If anything, Patti became indignant over his thinking that purging was "just a choice" and that she was doing this to herself on purpose. But as she was coming out of a sleepy fog, she overheard him recommending that her partner might want to bring in a priest to give last rites. Although a "cafeteria Catholic," who was very selective about what aspects of the Catholic church she agreed with, Patti felt strongly about the sacraments. "But extreme unction is for the elderly and the infirm," she thought. Then it dawned on her: "I really might die from this."

Until she heard the words "last rites," Patti had believed she was bulletproof—that somehow her body would keep bouncing back from the repeated insults of purging disorder. She had noticed that, as she got older, she wasn't bouncing back quite as quickly. A trip to the ER for fluids could put her out of commission for a week, whereas when she was younger she'd be back at work the next day.

When she woke up the next morning, alive, Patti thanked God for giving her another chance and vowed to her partner that she would truly dedicate herself to recovery—for her sake and for the sake of their relationship.

Rarely do dire warnings like those from Patti's physician get through the armor of eating disorders. The pervasive avoidance of emotion and false sense of invulnerability conferred by the eating disorder often render such threats impotent. Death is something that happens to those other people, but not to you. In Patti's case, it was digging deep into the trenches of her religious upbringing and knowledge about last rites that jolted her into awareness of just how serious her condition had become. Occasionally, seemingly random but deeply meaningful events can hook into a hidden drive for wellness and life and pull people onto a recovery path.

Spirituality

Spirituality is a motivator that we are far too hesitant to discuss, which is unfortunate because it can be an enormously powerful force in recovery. Spirituality offers another avenue to remove the focus from the self or the disorder and help keep the patient's focus outward. In *Restoring Our Bodies, Reclaiming Our Lives: Guidance and Reflections on Recovery from Eating Disorders*, edited by Aimee Liu, psychologist Josie Geller shares, "Finding a higher purpose is often associated with feeling less distress, more confidence, less preoccupation with body shape and weight, and greater openness to embarking on change."[1]

Peter Maffly-Kipp, clinical chaplain with the University of North Carolina's Center of Excellence for Eating Disorders, makes the following observation about spirituality and midlife eating disorders. "One of the things I have noticed is that someone who enters midlife with anorexia has really lost contact with their spiritual selves. They are often 'religious,' but in a distorted way that tends to be short on forgiveness, redemption, or grace (especially for themselves), and long on judgment and unworthiness. Kierkegaard called this the 'Sickness unto Death,' and said the lowest form of despair in a person involved a deep longing to be anyone but themselves (such that they are unable to recognize themselves)."

Peter works with adult patients to develop a more compassionate spirituality, which they can weave into their recovery matrix. Individuals with eating disorders can be extremely self-punishing, and the last thing they need is a punishing God in the mix. Developing a more nonjudgmental, accepting, and redemptive spirituality can be a gateway to developing those more gracious attitudes toward themselves.

A Life Without Self-Loathing (aka I Deserve to Recover)

"I don't deserve to take up space in the world. I don't deserve to be happy. I don't deserve to recover. I don't deserve to eat."

These comments are deeply intertwined with the self-loathing and self-punishing facets of eating disorders. Lucia, a woman in her mid-thirties with anorexia nervosa, always, without fail, stopped her therapy session after forty-nine minutes and told me, her therapist, that our time was up. Anything that happens that regularly in therapy has meaning, but the question was how best to address this. One day, she was very tired after a terrible night's sleep, and she let her guard down as she was discussing a very emotional topic. She missed her cue, and we went overtime. When she glanced at the clock and realized this, Lucia was horrified at having taken up so much of my time. She rapidly packed up her things and left and later sent me an e-mail apologizing and hoping she had not inconvenienced the patients who came after her. This incident became fodder for many sessions to come and illustrated that Lucia did not feel worthy of taking up any more of my time than she paid for. She would sit folded up on a chair not taking up space. She used very few words, not wanting to overfill the world with her own words. She had a core belief that she deserved less of everything than others and was mortified at the prospect of ever seeming selfish.

At the core of Lucia's behavior was a deep sense of self-loathing and self-punishment and an inability to see anything positive about who she was in the world. Working through this core belief can liberate patients, allowing them to recognize that they deserve to be healthy as much as anyone else does. Moreover, it lets them be okay with admitting they deserve the right to be healthy and happy. The self-punishing nature of eating disorders can take on religious overtones in those who believe that there is something fundamentally evil about them that renders them undeserving of time, love, and attention. Helping them to absolve themselves of this belief can be an important stepping-stone to and facilitator of recovery. For Lucia, it was allowing herself to believe that I truly cared about her—that it wasn't just me doing my job.

A New Identity

For twenty years, Abby's identity was her eating disorder. Throughout college, she was "the one with anorexia." After graduation, she got married and had a child (despite not menstruating), and she knew she was the topic of conversation of the other mothers in the neighborhood. She explained, "Wherever I went, whenever I was introduced to someone new, when I walked into church, when I went to the neighborhood pool, I knew that in everyone's minds they were saying, 'That's Abigail Smith . . . the woman with anorexia.' Maybe they didn't say it out loud, but when I walked away, they'd whisper, 'Yes, that's her.' People didn't invite us over for dinner; they always edited any comments about food and assumed—perhaps correctly—that I would disapprove of what they were eating. 'We're going to just stop and get fast food for dinner. Oh, Abby, I know you wouldn't approve.' Whenever I went running in the neighborhood, I knew they were just wondering when I was going to keel over and die."

Abby knew that, even once she gained weight and recovered from her eating disorder, it was still going to take a long time to change those perceptions. She wondered what people were going to say about her instead of "She's the woman with anorexia." During her recovery journey, she wasn't sure she even had an identity outside of her eating disorder: She had become her anorexia. The hardest thing for her to deal with was when people made comments about her new look. "You look so healthy." "You're glowing." "You look so much better." "Glad you've put on some weight." "It's good to see some meat on your bones." On some level, every one of these comments made her want to go out and run ten miles, but Abby resisted the temptation and reminded herself over and over again that people don't have a script about what to say when someone recovers from anorexia nervosa. As unfortunate as some of the comments might be, they were all well-meaning. Abby set out to craft a new epithet for herself as she rebuilt her post-anorexia identity. She started a nonprofit organization that collected and distributed food to underprivileged families in her community. Her husband thought it was ironic that someone who had been starving for so long threw herself into feeding people who did not have enough food, but she found it to be the perfect vehicle for healing and "giving back." After five years of directing the nonprofit and speaking about it in the community, now when she went to the pool, people would say, "That's Abigail, the director of Thoughtful Food."

Contribution

Rachel was reading the newspaper one Saturday morning and saw an article about people in her community raising funds to help a local family that had lost everything in a fire. She had heard about this family and was distressed by their story, but she'd done nothing about it. Rachel asked herself why she hadn't done anything, yet these other families were spending their weekends gathering provisions, raising funds, and doing everything within their power to help this family rebuild their lives. She realized that it was because she was spending her weekends at drive-throughs and doughnut shops, drowning her own troubles, and the troubles of the world, in food. In fact, she recalled that she'd been in the middle of a binge in her car when she had first heard this family's story on the radio. But instead of doing something about it at the time, she had sat there eating. This realization was a real turning point for Rachel, as she developed insight into the fact that her eating disorder had completely robbed her of the opportunity to contribute to her community. Before she developed BED, she had led a reading group, volunteered at the local thrift store, and run a youth group at her temple—but that all had stopped when her eating disorder had gone into full swing. Rachel felt as if BED had robbed meaning from her life.

For some people, this kind of an "aha" moment can catapult them into rejoining their communities and fixing their gaze more outward than inward. Rachel, like many patients, looked back on her disordered eating days and, with shame in her voice, acknowledged how it had been "all about her." She was clear that her eating disorder was enormously self-centered and had held her back from being a full participant in the world.

Choose Happiness

In looking back over twenty years of an eating disorder, Esther recalled, "Happiness just wasn't on my radar screen." Even as a young, overweight girl, when her friends were discussing what would make them happy, she just didn't think happiness was a goal she could allow herself to have. Esther's only goals were weight goals; happiness was for other people, for thin people. So she spent the next twenty years simply "going through the motions." She had a marriage, a career, and a dog, but her only real relationship was with food. This was not apparent from the outside, since Esther seemed enormously competent and successful, contributed to her community, and had a reasonably comfortable marriage. On the inside, however, she felt nothing. Her therapist asked her what brought happiness to her life, and she literally had no answer. In fact, she felt as if she did not have the right to be happy because she was fat. Esther firmly believed that fat and happy were incompatible. She had given up on fighting the fat and, after countless diets, had reconciled herself to the fact that she would always be large; but with that reconciliation had come the complete relinquishment of ever being happy.

Esther's therapist challenged her basic assumption that one is not entitled to be happy if one is large, a core belief that Esther had held since she was about seven years old. Her therapy revolved around this central assertion, and for years, they worked together unpacking how that belief had become so fixed in her mind. Gradually, Esther began to ease the reins and wonder whether it was still possible, even at age fifty, to allow herself to experience happiness. Together, she and her therapist introduced small experiences of pleasure and joy, really working to develop a new range of emotional experiences that Esther had never allowed herself to feel. Seemingly minor things she would have typically overlooked, such as a blooming flower, a blue sky, a kind act, or someone's smile, all started to accumulate into a library of positive emotions for her, which allowed Esther to gradually become more comfortable with having allowed herself to choose happiness.

Just because eating disorders are in part caused by biology does not mean that active choice is not involved in recovery. We constantly face decision nodes during the course of each and every day. In Esther's case, she had to choose to allow herself to be happy; no therapist could force this on her. Making active choices in the direction of health is what paves the path to recovery.

AWARENESS AND ACTION

These examples are only a subset of motivators for recovery, and everyone's library of motivators has to be uniquely tailored to his or her personal circumstances. Develop your own library and make it concrete. Whether you catalog it electronically or make an actual "recovery box," capture your thoughts and rectify them. A resourceful patient of mine repurposed a plastic container that her new mouse came in to be her recovery toolbox. She created her own list of motivators for the toolbox and crafted little symbols for each one. Inspired by the Noun Project (www.thenoun project.com), she found that symbols rather than words spoke to her "right brain," tapping into the emotional—rather than purely intellectual—reasons she wanted to recover. Plus, if anyone was to find her box, they would have no clue that it was a recovery toolbox since it was just an odd collection of symbols! Find a way to create your own recovery resource and tailor it especially for you. Bring it out whenever you need a motivation boost and continue to build it. Your recovery toolbox should be an organic tool that grows and expands as your journey progresses.

CHAPTER 11

Finding Compassionate Care

Once you have committed to seeking help for your eating disorder, the first steps can be quite bewildering. Many variables go into decisions about where to seek treatment and how to find the kind of treatment that is right for you. This chapter dissects the treatment process into several important components, weighs the pros and cons of various approaches, and highlights pitfalls that can complicate finding compassionate care. The type and level of care you may be seeking will vary considerably based on what type of eating disorder you have, how severe your disorder is, and the availability of treatment in your area. However, some principles in treatment seeking cut across disorders and severity, and we will review those first.

What Is Evidence-Based Treatment?
The term "evidence-based treatment" is heard often in advocacy circles, but this is not a term that is familiar to most people. When you visit your primary care physician, you make an implicit assumption that she or he keeps up with continuing medical education requirements, stays on top of the latest scientific literature, attends relevant conferences and presentations, and practices medicine according to the best scientific and medical evidence. You would not be pleased to discover that he or she did not keep up with the latest medical news and was treating an ailment of yours with an outdated inter-

vention or a treatment that had never been shown to be effective. It is, after all, your health and your life at stake.

You are entitled to these same expectations when it comes to the treatment of eating disorders. You want to be assured that your therapist or treatment team are well trained, have experience in the treatment of eating disorders, and are providing you with clinical care that is up to contemporary standards and based on the latest evidence for effective treatment protocols.

This issue can become complicated, however, because the evidence base for treating some eating disorders in midlife is meager. For example, although we have a fair bit of evidence about treatment for bulimia nervosa and BED in midlife (because most of the clinical trials included individuals of broad age ranges with these disorders), we know much less about the treatment of anorexia nervosa in this age group. Further complicating the picture, many of the clinical trials have included mostly women and mostly Caucasian participants. Thus, the extent to which even the evidence-based treatments are effective in men, as well as in people from racial and ethnic minority groups, remains unknown. Just admitting to having an eating disorder can encounter barriers. One African-American man recalled raising the idea he might have anorexia with his African-American male physician, who responded, "It must be something else, that doesn't happen to us."

It can be challenging for patients and caretakers to judge which programs or therapists provide evidence-based treatment. Unfortunately, the nature of the U.S. health care system and the absence of a strong evidence base open the door to marketing of programs and unchecked claims about success. The treatment of eating disorders is a business—a Big business—and people with eating disorders and their family members are a vulnerable market. Unfortunately, when you or a loved one is ill and desperate, it is not the easiest time to engage your critical thinking skills and be skeptical when programs are offering you hope.

Jed, the husband of a thirty-seven-year-old woman with anorexia nervosa, had done an enormous amount of research on programs around the country before choosing a treatment center for his wife. He was diligent, asked smart questions, and weighed the information he got against what he knew about anorexia nervosa. Jed recalled, "So as I called around, I heard all sorts of claims—one program boasted a ninety-eight-percent cure rate, another that they were the most successful program in the country, another employed gourmet chefs to prepare meals, and several emphasized the importance of equine therapy in recovery." He continued, "First off, as far as I know, there is no 'cure' for anorexia nervosa. Second, no study I have ever heard of had a ninety-eight-percent positive outcome. Third, how could they compare themselves to the other programs around the country without any data to back up their claims? Fourth, I had taken her to all the best restaurants with all the best chefs thinking that something would convince her to eat. If gourmet food fixed anorexia, she'd be fine by now. And as far as horses go . . . she'd break her pelvis if she rode a horse!" His emotions took over as he exclaimed, "I was angry. I felt marketed to. I was trying to seek care for my wife who was dying before my very eyes, and all they could see were dollar signs."

It is also important to consider what evidence-based treatment is not. Evidence-based treatment does not mean that the treatment works for everyone. It simply means that it has been shown in rigorous investigations to work better than no treatment at all, to work better than a placebo treatment, or to work better than another treatment that it was compared to. The results are based only on the group of people who are tested, and individuals within those groups may respond differently to a given treatment (see figure on next page). I have heard patients and partners lament the fact that an evidence-based treat-

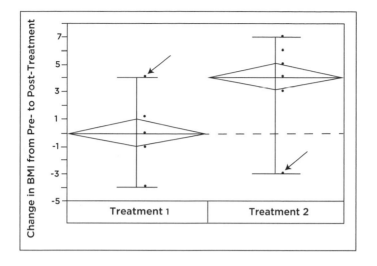

*Looking at BMI change as an outcome, Treatment 2 clearly outperforms
Treatment 1, as the average change in BMI is higher in the people
who received Treatment 2. However, one patient in Treatment 1
responded very well, and one patient in Treatment 2 responded
very poorly. Evidence-based treatment does not mean that one treatment
works for all individuals.*

ment didn't work for them, followed by concern that there was
something wrong with them because the treatment hadn't been
effective. This is precisely why we need a broader evidence base.

For example, if you go to your physician with high blood
pressure, chances are good that she will start with trying to
modify your diet and exercise patterns. If that is not effective
in bringing your blood pressure down, she may try a medication. If that medication doesn't work well, or if you have intolerable side effects, she'll reach into her little black bag and
find another medication to try—until she finds the medication
that is right for you. The same principle holds with the treatment of eating disorders. Just because one approach does not

work for you at a certain point in time, it does not mean that it will not work for you at a later point in time or that there is not another treatment that will work well for you. Sometimes effective treatment is a series of trial-and-error experiments until the correct fit is found.

There are both similarities and differences in the treatment options that are available and have been shown to be effective for the various eating disorders. In order to present the broadest picture of available interventions, we will cover some basics to consider when selecting a program. Then we will focus on several dimensions: levels of care, selecting providers and programs, psychotherapies, and medications. After reviewing the complete landscape of these dimensions, we will delve disorder by disorder into the evidence base to describe, in depth, what the science has revealed to us about their efficacy.

Levels of Care
There are five basic levels of care for the treatment of eating disorders. Not every level is available in every country, and the types of treatment offered are influenced by the nature of the health care system. The highest level of care is inpatient treatment, which involves around-the-clock supervision in a hospital and can be in a medical or psychiatric unit of a general or more specialized facility. Typically, inpatient care is most common for anorexia nervosa and generally occurs during the renourishment and weight restoration phase, or if a patient has deteriorated physically or psychologically at some point during the course of recovery. It may also be appropriate for individuals with bulimia nervosa who are medically unstable, or whose disorder simply cannot be controlled at a lower level of care. Inpatient treatment can occur on a medical ward if a patient is medically compromised or of there are no other services available for short-term medically supervised renourishment. If general psychiatric inpatient facilities or a medical-psychiatry unit are available, then more prolonged treatment might occur there for longer renour-

ishment and to address the psychological aspects of the eating disorders, as well as any psychiatric comorbidities, such as depression or anxiety. Inpatient programs benefit from having additional medical care and consultation available due to their close proximity to other hospital departments.

When available, the preferred inpatient environment is a specialty eating disorders service. In such a service, staff are trained and dedicated to the treatment of eating disorders, and all or most patients on the service are suffering from an eating disorder. A multidisciplinary team provides clinical care and specialized programming that addresses the eating disorder from medical, psychological, family, and dietary perspectives.

Residential programs also involve full-time, around-the-clock care but are in noninstitutional settings. These generally provide more luxurious settings, and they may not have the extensive medical backup seen in inpatient programs. Stays can be longer, and treatment costs can be high. Residential programs are typically characterized by specific offerings, such as a particular therapeutic orientation or the nature of the setting (e.g., desert, mountains, rural).

Partial hospitalization is the step between inpatient and outpatient treatment. It can serve as a step-down treatment after individuals have completed inpatient treatment, or as a higher level of care beyond outpatient if inpatient is not warranted. Typically, a partial hospitalization program includes programming from morning through evening, covering all mealtimes. Patients are then free to spend the evenings and weekends at home. Partial hospitalization provides the structure of full-day programming while introducing the real-world challenges faced when returning home. Successes and challenges can then be quickly processed the next day. Partial hospitalization provides an important buffer between inpatient and outpatient treatment, given that jumping from around-the-clock care to a few hours a week of outpatient therapy can feel like jumping off a cliff. Partial hospitalization softens the transition and allows for plenty of practice and exposure to the challenges of the outside world before graduating to outpatient.

Intensive outpatient treatment is not universally available, but generally refers to an outpatient program that takes place for a couple of hours per day between three to five days per week. One example would be an evening program from five to eight P.M., which can be ideal for individuals in midlife who have full-time jobs during the day. Intensive outpatient programs also include structured group programming, typically a shared meal, and individual care by a physician and therapist. They can serve as another step-down treatment after partial hospitalization or as a step-up from once-a-week outpatient therapy to provide additional structure and support.

Outpatient treatment can include a range of interventions, including medication management with a physician or nurse practitioner, individual therapy, group therapy, family-based therapy, dietary counseling, and couple-based therapy. Outpatient therapy is appropriate for less severe presentations, for people who are stepping down from higher levels of care, when other options aren't available in the community for a patient who is medically stable, and for maintenance treatment.

Treatment Team: Or, Recovery May Take a Village
For all eating disorders, treatment is often provided by more than one clinician. The multidisciplinary team approach is most common in the treatment of anorexia nervosa but may be used in varying degrees to treat other eating disorders. For all disorders, especially patients in midlife, a thorough medical examination is strongly recommended as the starting point. As we age, the number of medical conditions that could masquerade as eating disorders increases (e.g., cancer, tumors, thyroid disease). Moreover, older bodies are less resilient to the damaging effects of an eating disorder, so they require closer medical observation.

For the treatment of anorexia nervosa, a comprehensive

team could include some combination of the following: 1) a primary care physician to monitor laboratory values and other medical problems; 2) a psychiatrist to manage any psychotropic medications that may be prescribed, and to interface with the primary care physician; 3) a primary therapist (e.g., psychologist, social worker, or counselor) with special expertise in providing psychotherapy for eating disorders; 4) a registered dietitian to work on meal planning and collaboratively set weight-gain goals; and, if the patient is in a relationship, 5) a couple therapist. The most important feature of any treatment team is communication. With this many providers, it is essential that they all be on the same page with regard to treatment goals and benchmarks. Having one clinician serve as the quarterback can ensure that communication continues smoothly across the course of treatment and that the patient and caregivers are receiving consistent messages from the entire team. This can also prevent any splitting that the eating disorder might attempt; for example, trying to negotiate a lower weight-gain goal with the weakest link on the team. During inpatient, residential, or partial hospitalization treatment, other team members may also contribute to care, including specialized nursing staff, social workers, family therapists, occupational therapists, recreational therapists, physical therapists, and chaplains. Consultation with other medical specialists (e.g., gastroenterology, cardiology, nephrology) may also occur as needed.

For bulimia nervosa and BED, treatment teams tend to be smaller and consist of a therapist skilled in the treatment of eating disorders and either a primary care physician or psychiatrist. Dietitians are extremely valuable in the treatment of both of these disorders; unfortunately, insurance coverage for dietary counseling is often hard to come by. If you can, it is worth paying out of pocket for as many sessions as you can afford. Dietitians can assist with meal planning, dietary diversity, portion evaluation, and dealing with both nutritional and emotional aspects of developing healthy eating patterns.

Selecting a Therapist

Let's place the task of selecting a therapist in context. You are about to choose someone with whom you are going to share an enormous number of details about your life, your thoughts, and your feelings. You are selecting someone to help guide and support you through a potentially rocky and nonlinear path of recovery. You are selecting someone who you need to trust to help you make wise decisions about your health and your health care. You are selecting someone with whom you may work for several years. As if those factors aren't enough, you are likely going to be paying him or her a considerable amount of money.

So, first and foremost, you want the therapist to have appropriate credentials and be professional. Therapists should be completely forthcoming about their training and experience with eating disorders, but it is your responsibility to ask. If you were having knee replacement surgery, you would ask the surgeon how many knee replacement operations she or he had performed. Same thing with eating disorders treatment: you have a right to know how many cases of eating disorders the therapist has treated. Many providers simply list an array of disorders on their competency checklists, and your insurance company may send you to someone who is in-network but who saw just one eating disorders patient during his or her clinical internship. Your insurance company's provider list is not always the best place to start for an eating disorders referral. I had a patient come to me recently with a list from her insurance company of "experts" who were in-network and who treat eating disorders, and I didn't recognize one of them. Furthermore, none of their names showed up on any of my professional referral lists! If there is no one in network who has experience in eating disorders, get on the phone and talk with someone in your insurance company.

Of course, there are financial, insurance, and geographic constraints that will influence your selection of a therapist. Even when considering those critical factors, you must ad-

dress the issue of "fit." When we asked people who had suffered from anorexia nervosa in the past what the most
important factor was in their recovery, their first response was
"relationships." That could be a relationship with a loved one or
a therapist, but relationships were the number-one factor that
they felt contributed to their recovery. Therapy is a relationship.
It is a special kind of relationship, with basic parameters that
are different from those of a friendship, but it is critical to attend carefully to whether you feel that you will be able to develop a therapeutic relationship with your prospective therapist.

You may have received a referral for a therapist from an
eating disorders program or organization, but the truth is, few
of us professionals ever see or hear our colleagues conducting a
psychotherapy session. Unless we have supervised them in some
capacity, we can only infer how they are as therapists from what
they are like as people, what we know they know about eating
disorders from conversations, and what their patients report.
The best barometer of therapeutic fit is your own intuition.

Unfortunately, it is not always easy to trust your intuition
in these situations. Most people are a little—or even very—
nervous the first time they meet with a therapist. This makes
perfect sense. It is a logical and natural thing to feel. It is also
important, despite your nervousness, to pay attention to your
own perceptions of the interaction. Sometimes we might brush
off observations as not important, but sometimes the reactions
that pop into and then out of our heads are the most important
ones to pay attention to. There is no expectation that you commit to a therapist after your first session together. It is perfectly acceptable to talk with a few therapists on the phone or
face-to-face, evaluate your reactions to each, and then choose
the best fit for you.

In evaluating these initial meetings, ask yourself some
pointed questions. Did I feel comfortable? Did she seem to be
knowledgeable and confident? Was the therapist attentive and

focused on what I was saying? Did I feel listened to and under-
stood or was she not quite getting where I was coming from?
Did I like the room? Is this a place where I can spend time and
be myself? Was there anything that he did that raised red flags
(lots of checking the clock, yawning, looking out the window,
dozing off)? Did it feel like she genuinely cared about my well-
being? Did he feel trustworthy? Did I feel judged? Did she
"get" eating disorders? Was there anything else that I particularly liked or disliked about the experience?

Selecting a Program
Much like selecting a therapist, selecting a treatment program
has to take into consideration your severity of illness, financial
situation, geographic location, age and gender, and the fit between your personality and that of the program. In making
your decision, a wise starting point is to consider an important
document developed by the Academy for Eating Disorders in
2005 called the World Wide Charter for Action on Eating Disorders.[1] The charter addresses six primary directives:

1. Right to communication/partnership with health
   professionals.
2. Right to comprehensive assessment and treatment
   planning.
3. Right to accessible, high quality, fully funded,
   specialized care.
4. Right to respectful, fully informed, age-appropriate,
   safe levels of care.
5. Right of carers to be informed, valued, and re-
   spected as a treatment resource.
6. Right of carers to accessible, appropriate support
   and education resources.

Obviously, providers cannot guarantee fully funded care,
and as such, this remains an aspirational document. However,

the other core principles are entirely appropriate for patients and partners to expect as they seek treatment for an eating disorder.

The Psychotherapy Landscape

Before diving into the evidence base for the treatment of the various eating disorders, you need to wrap your head around the types of psychotherapy that either have been tested or are being used in the treatment of adults with eating disorders.

Even before you get to the point of being in a room with a therapist, there are a variety of self-help approaches for the treatment of some eating disorders. Although self-help is not recommended for the treatment of anorexia nervosa, in the United Kingdom, according to the national guidelines,[2] self-help is recommended as the first line of treatment for BED. As such, a number of books, workbooks, online programs, CD-ROMs, and smartphone apps have been developed to assist with the management of BED.[3] The majority of these focus heavily on self-monitoring of behaviors, thoughts, and feelings and use what is primarily a cognitive behavioral approach. Many of these approaches can also be used as an adjunct to treatment of anorexia and bulimia nervosa, but they are not recommended as the sole intervention.

Delving into the alphabet soup of acronyms for psychotherapeutic approaches, we start with cognitive behavioral therapy (CBT), which was originally developed for the treatment of depression.[4] The fundamental tenets of the CBT treatment model are that emotional and behavioral experiences are mediated by the way in which an individual cognitively processes information in a particular situation. Or, your thoughts drive your behaviors and feelings. You have different layers of thoughts. Perceptions and thoughts are on the surface and are your interface with experience; automatic thoughts run just beneath the surface and are often judgmental; and deeper and less accessible core beliefs are guiding principles or truths for an individual. The application of CBT to eating disorders rests on the principle that faulty cognitions about body shape, weight, eating, and personal control lead to and maintain the dysfunction in eating and weight. The treatment involves identifying, challenging, and replacing dyfunctional thoughts about food, eating, body shape, and weight, and thereby paving the way for healthier non-disordered behaviors.

Specialist supportive clinical management (SSCM) is a form of therapy that aims to mimic, as closely as possible, the kind of outpatient treatment offered for treating eating disorders in typical clinical practice.[5] SSCM combines features of sound clinical management and supportive psychotherapy. Within the SSCM framework, anorexia nervosa is conceptualized as a serious disorder that, regardless of its cause, is essentially maintained by insufficient and dysfunctional eating. SSCM views the adoption of healthy eating and restoration of weight to within a normal range as a fundamental core of treatment. Therefore, the major aim of SSCM is to assist the patient in establishing or reestablishing healthy eating patterns and a healthy weight by providing education and advice about anorexia nervosa and nutrition, as well as to support and encourage the patient in implementing this advice and making appropriate changes. If the mechanisms that maintain the disorder are addressed directly, it is hypothesized that the distressing symptoms, disability, and disruption associated with anorexia nervosa will be alleviated. SSCM recognizes that other factors invariably affect a patient's eating behavior and has the flexibility to deal with whatever topics the patient brings into the room.

Interpersonal psychotherapy (IPT) is a brief, time-limited psychotherapy that was initially developed for the treatment of depression,[6] and it has since been adapted for the treatment of bulimia nervosa,[7] anorexia nervosa,[8] and BED.[9] The theoretical underpinnings of IPT for eating disorders are that, regardless of the causes of the eating disorder, the current symptoms are "inextricably intertwined" with the patient's interpersonal relationships. The goals of the intervention are to decrease eating disorder symptoms and improve interpersonal functioning by enhancing communication skills in significant relationships. IPT focuses on one of four problem areas: interpersonal disputes, role transitions, abnormal grief, or interpersonal deficits.

Dialectical behavioral therapy (DBT) is an intensive system of therapy originally developed by Marsha M. Linehan, Ph.D., for the treatment of borderline personality disorder, a condition in which people have marked impulsivity and long-term patterns of unstable or turbulent emotions.[10] DBT combines CBT techniques for emotional regulation with therapeutic approaches rooted in Buddhist meditative practice to address distress tolerance, acceptance, and mindful awareness.

Motivational interviewing (MI) has its roots in addressing the ambivalence that problem drinkers experience engaging in treatment.[11] The explicit goal of MI is for the therapist to elicit behavior change by resolving ambivalence. MI acknowledges that patients enter treatment with varying degrees of readiness to change,[12] so the treatment approach focuses explicitly on the here and now and "meets patients where they're at." MI does not judge, but helps raise awareness of the value of choosing change and the consequences of not choosing change. MI is geared toward enhancing motivation to change via the expression of empathy, exploring the discrepancy between how life currently is and how the patient desires it to be, rolling with resistance (rather than confronting inertia), and supporting the patient's self-efficacy to choose change.

Acceptance and commitment therapy (ACT) is a popular acceptance-based model of CBT that emphasizes changing behaviors rather than altering internal experiences.[13] The goal of ACT is to help patients consistently choose to act effectively through concrete behaviors defined by their values, even in the presence of difficult or disruptive "private" (cognitive or psychological) events. ACT also describes what takes place in therapy: accept the effects of life's hardships, choose directional values, and take action. The developers describe six core processes of ACT: acceptance, cognitive defusion, being present, self as context, valuing, and committed action. Acceptance refers to letting your feelings and thoughts happen without having to act on them. Cognitive defusion techniques are aimed at changing how you relate to, and interact with, your thoughts in order to decrease their unhelpful functions. Being present refers to remaining aware of the here and now. Self as context is a form of self-observation that acknowledges your consistency across time. Valuing encourages you to focus on what is important to your true self. And, finally, committed action refers to setting goals consistent with your values and carrying them out.

Uniting Couples (in the treatment of) Anorexia Nervosa (UCAN) is a couple-based intervention that grew from the awareness that family-based therapy is the evidence-based treatment of choice for youth with anorexia nervosa, yet none of the tested interventions for anorexia nervosa in adults leveraged family support.[14] UCAN is a form of cognitive behavioral couple therapy and is based on the premise that, although one member of the couple has anorexia nervosa, the disorder occurs in an interpersonal and social context. For married patients or those in a committed relationship, the partner is a central part of their social environment and, thus, can contribute to improvement—or conversely, may help maintain or even exacerbate the eating disorder. While many partners want to help, they often don't know how to do so and may unknowingly make the situation worse. UCAN uses a three-phase approach. The initial phase of treatment focuses on understanding the couple's experience with the eating disorder, educating the couple about the disorder and recovery process, and then teaching them effective communication skills. Creating a shared understanding of the eating disorder sets the stage for a greater sense of teamwork and leads to improved communication and problem-solving skills. In the second phase, the couple is guided through the areas of the eating disorder they find most challenging, including purging, binge eating, and secrecy. They learn to use their communication skills to respond to these challenges—as a team. Then, the treatment team broadens the focus to include body image and sexual issues as they relate to the eating disorder. The focus on body image provides a natural approach to the couple's physical relationship, and the couple is helped to develop healthier patterns appropriate for them. The final phase brings treatment to a close by discussing ways to prevent relapse and the next steps for the couple after the treatment ends. The couple learns to differentiate slips from relapses and learns ways to effectively respond to each if they do occur. UCAN is being adapted for treatment of other eating disorders as well.

Although you may encounter many additional acronyms when exploring treatments for an eating disorder, these are the ones that currently form the basis of the evidence base for eating disorders treatment and the ones that will be emphasized as we review treatments disorder by disorder.

It is worth mentioning that many therapists in private practice do not adhere to just one of these approaches. They may combine elements from various therapies to create their own eclectic or integrative and flexible style. This has both pluses (allows for greater flexibility with a range of patients) and minuses (it strays from the evidence base and we don't really know what the effects of this type of flexibility are on outcome). Most important is that the therapist have sound training in one or more of the approaches and that his or her eclecticism be truly a flexible utilization of evidence-based approaches, rather than a shoot-from-the-hip uninformed or generic approach.

The Pharmacotherapy Landscape

Many medications have been tested in the treatment of anorexia nervosa, bulimia nervosa, and BED, and their names and categories can be even more bewildering than the psychotherapy acronyms. To simplify matters, we'll review them by class. The first group of medications that have been tried are the antidepressants. There are older trials of the first-generation antidepressants, like tricyclic antidepressants and monoamine oxidase inhibitors, which can be distinguished from the "second-generation antidepressants" such as serotonin and norepinephrine reuptake inhibitors (SNRIs) and selective serotonin reuptake inhibitors (SSRIs). Other types of medications that have been studied for eating disorder treatment include anticonvulsant medications, antianxiety medications, and antipsychotic medications, as well as medications that are primarily directed toward appetite control, appetite stimulation, or weight loss. These classes of medications will be reviewed below as we explore pharmacologic approaches to the treatment of each disorder.

Treatment for Anorexia Nervosa

Goals of Inpatient Treatment. The goals of inpatient treatment are generally to achieve renourishment and begin the psychological work associated with recovery from anorexia nervosa. In addition, medical stabilization, nutritional rehabilitation and reeducation, treatment of comorbid conditions (such as depression or substance abuse), and family education, support, and therapy are all important aspects of inpatient treatment.

The American Psychiatric Association Working Group on Eating Disorders recommends hospitalization for individuals below 75 percent of ideal body weight,[15] although weight should not be the only parameter to be considered in determining which level of care is most appropriate. Other factors that may warrant inpatient care include serious medical complications, a past suicide attempt or suicide plan, unsuccessful weight gain in outpatient or partial hospitalization treatment, the presence of comorbid conditions, significant impairment to roles at home and/or work, poor psychosocial support, if the patient is pregnant and struggling, and if lower levels of care aren't available. Ideally, patients would remain inpatient until they reach 90 to 95 percent of ideal body weight. In fact, the likelihood of a revolving door (readmission) goes down the closer an individual is to a healthy weight.

The average length of inpatient stay for anorexia nervosa in the United States is about twenty-six days.[16] Although this may sound like a long time, it is substantially shorter than the averages in other countries, including New Zealand (seventy-two days)[17] and throughout Europe, where inpatient stays range from 62.3 days (Czech Republic) to 197.4 days (the Netherlands).[18] The reason for such lengthy treatment is that renourishment cannot be achieved overnight. At times, when insurance companies are pressuring medical providers to force discharge of a patient prematurely, one gets the sense that the insurance companies just want the doctors to magically "reinflate" people with anorexia nervosa and get them back on the road. People aren't tires, and every body responds differently to the renourishment process.

Gaining weight too quickly can be associated with "refeeding syndrome," which is rare but potentially fatal.[19] Rapid refeeding can result in dangerous shifts in fluids, electrolytes, and metabolism that can affect basically every bodily organ. A safer approach is based on judicious, sequential planned caloric increases, requiring daily management to respond to potential complications such as liver inflammation and hypoglycemia. Individuals with anorexia nervosa often have delayed gastric transit time and other types of digestive distress that make rapid refeeding distressing and uncomfortable, and renourishment is a highly anxiety-provoking phase of treatment.[20] When not done skillfully and sensitively, it can be traumatizing; and it can also invite a transition to bulimia if the patient is encouraged to "eat his or her way out of the hospital," only to be discharged and lose weight again.

Goals of Residential Treatment. In the treatment of anorexia nervosa, the goals of residential treatment are to re-nourish, to work on the psychological aspects of the disorder (usually in a community setting), and to get the patient to the point where she or he is prepared to return to the challenges of home. Longer stays can facilitate more gradual recovery, but costs can also pose substantial financial burden to patients and families.

Goals of Partial Hospitalization Treatment. For anorexia nervosa, the partial hospitalization bridge can be a time for additional weight gain or stabilization of weight gained during inpatient or residential treatment. More important, partial hospitalization takes the psychological aspect of recovery one step farther, with additional and more intensive psychotherapy groups and greater focus on maintaining treatment gains and preventing relapse. In partial hospitalization, patients have greater autonomy in meal planning and eating. Given that patients return home during evenings and weekends, partial hospitalization also allows for more exposure-based treatment. Time away from the hospital means confrontations with real-world challenges. Patients can practice at restaurants, with families, and at social events and then process their successes and challenges when they are back with the team. Returning to the hospital after such encounters uses these challenges, and the patient's response to them as grist for the therapeutic mill and to bolster the next stages of recovery. Partial hospitalization also focuses strongly on relapse prevention strategies and on preparation for stepping down to a less intensive level of care.

Goals of Outpatient Treatment. Outpatient treatment is appropriate for less severe cases of anorexia nervosa when patients are medically stable, and for individuals stepping down from inpatient (if partial hospitalization is not available), residential, or partial hospitalization treatment. It can also be an important component of treatment of individuals with chronic anorexia. Outpatient treatment is where recovery from anorexia nervosa is consolidated. In youth, outpatient treatment in the form of family therapy may be the cornerstone of recovery. For midlife patients with eating disorders, outpatient treatment is also central, but it may come in many forms. Individual treatment may be augmented by therapy groups and, where available and appropriate to the situation, by couple-based therapy or family therapy. Outpatient treatment can also include medical monitoring by a primary care physician and/or psychiatrist.

Psychotherapy. When we look at the types of psychotherapy that have been shown to be effective in the treatment of adult anorexia nervosa, we are struck by the paucity of literature. Much of the work on anorexia nervosa has been conducted on youth. We have some evidence that CBT may reduce relapse risk for adults with anorexia nervosa after they have gained weight in the hospital.[21] However, we know less about which psychotherapeutic interventions are effective when the patients are actively ill and underweight. One study that we conducted in New Zealand suggested that SSCM, as described previously, fared somewhat better than CBT,[22] and more recently, we have been continuously impressed with the ability of UCAN, the couple-based intervention, to keep patients in treatment and to support recovery by leveraging the power of a couple's relationship to fight anorexia as a team.[23]

Regardless of the type of therapy an individual with midlife anorexia nervosa receives, outpatient treatment should always be geared toward weight gain or continued weight stabilization at as close to 100 percent of ideal body weight as possible and toward improving psychological functioning. Many patients hover at lower weights for years in a state of partial recovery, increasing the risk of relapse. Ongoing medical monitoring and medication management is important, as medical conditions and medication effectiveness can change during the course of recovery with changing weight. Family members and partners continue to benefit from involvement in treatment during the outpatient phase. Even after patients have reached the point of discharge from outpatient treatment, booster sessions or follow-up appointments may be scheduled to ensure recovery remains on track.

Medications. The literature regarding medication treatments for anorexia nervosa is sparse and inconclusive.[24] There are no FDA-approved medications for the treatment of anorexia nervosa, and there are no clinical trials that have offered much promise. Many medications are prescribed off-label, and patients and practitioners do see benefit from some medications. There is, however, no magic pill to treat anorexia nervosa.

In fact, many medications are ineffective in low-weight individuals who are undernourished. There are some data to suggest that second-generation antidepressants such as fluoxetine (Prozac) can be effective in managing symptoms of anxiety and depression and assisting with weight maintenance after weight has been restored. In addition, some studies suggest that atypical antipsychotic medication can help reduce agitation and excessive physical activity, and some patients report that the renourishment process is more tolerable when they are taking atypical antipsychotic medications.[25]

INVOLUNTARY COMMITMENT

Although entering treatment voluntarily is always preferred, when individuals with eating disorders cannot care for themselves at home, or if they become a danger to themselves or others, they may have to be institutionalized against their will using civil commitment procedures. Commitment is a state-initiated procedure that forces involuntary treatment on people who are judged to be mentally ill and to present a danger to themselves (including the inability to care for themselves) or others,[26] and who refuse to participate in treatment voluntarily.

Involuntary treatment for eating disorders is most commonly prescribed for those suffering from anorexia nervosa, consent for which may be obtained through legal means or the threat of legal action. Laws vary across national borders, and within the United States from state to state. Patients' responses to commitment are complex.[27] In interviews with twenty-nine women, researchers report, "Patients with anorexia nervosa experience high levels of 'perceived coercion'—that is, the perception that they are being coerced whether or not formal mechanisms are used." Patients describe feeling pressure to accept seemingly "voluntary" treatment, though they acknowledge that using compulsive treatment, whether via legal means or informal coercion from their family or treatment team, may be called for in life-threatening cases (and are often grateful, in hindsight, that such actions were taken). The authors of these studies also recognize that the combination of low body weight, poor physical condition, and cognitive impairment may put patients in a position where they are unable to make decisions for themselves, and that "no one should die from a treatable disorder"—that the most important consideration is sustaining life.

That being said, in interviews, patients reported that they experience legal commitment for treatment as stigmatizing, and they worried about loss of personal freedom and control over the terms of their treatment. They also were less supportive of compulsory treatment when the case was not life-threatening, going so far as to argue that it was counterproductive to achieving recovery, which "required some degree of consent and cooperation" from the patient, and could do more harm than good. Interestingly, patients were less resentful about the commitment itself and more resentful at feeling "dismissed, belittled, or punitively treated . . . and being stripped of their individuality." Relationships, particularly those with parents and clinicians, were cited as a key mediator of outcomes, with trusting relationships playing a role in willingness to seek treatment or acceptance of forced treatment.[28]

The complexity of commitment from the patient's perspective is best captured by an eloquent former patient looking back on a hospitalization in which I saw no option but to recommend civil commitment. She was committed, and eventually she chose to remain in treatment voluntarily. Looking back on the experience, she said to me, "I hated you for having me committed, but you saved my life, so, thank you."

Treatment for Bulimia Nervosa

Goals of Inpatient, Residential, Partial Hospitalization, and Outpatient Treatment. In today's world, inpatient treatment for bulimia nervosa is rarely more than a short stay for medical stabilization. Few insurance companies will consider long-term inpatient hospitalization for bulimia nervosa. When a higher level of care is required, individuals with bulimia nervosa are more likely to be approved for residential or partial hospitalization; however, if higher levels of care are not supported by their insurance companies, these treatments have to be paid for out of pocket. Either way, the goals of inpatient hospitalization for bulimia nervosa are generally medical stabilization and, if possible, disrupting the entrenched binge-purge cycle. Residential and partial hospitalization are also geared toward interrupting the binge-purge cycle, normalizing meals and snacks, addressing any comorbid conditions, and dealing with the psychological components of the disorder. Partial hospitalization allows patients to experience the relative safety of the program during the day, but face the challenges of the outside world during evenings and weekends. Being able to go home and face those challenges without binge eating or purging are important experiences to have before stepping down to outpatient treatment. Succumbing to an urge to binge or purge while still in partial hospitalization allows the patient the opportunity to process the slip with staff and develop plans for the next evening or weekend. Most treatment for bulimia nervosa is delivered in outpatient settings, where the goals are abstinence from binge eating and purging, normalization of meals, addressing comorbid conditions, and dealing with the psychological components of the disorder.

Psychotherapy. Psychotherapy remains the treatment of choice for bulimia nervosa,[29] particularly CBT, which can be delivered either one-on-one with a therapist or in a group setting. Novel treatments incorporating technology are also exploring delivery of CBT via the Internet and using smartphone apps. Whatever the avenue of delivery, CBT is effective in reducing or eliminating binge eating and purging in around two thirds of patients with bulimia nervosa. Other types of psychotherapy, including IPT and DBT, have been shown to benefit patients, but the evidence is most robust for CBT. Psychotherapy can be delivered alone or in conjunction with medications, which can help jump-start treatment by reducing binge eating and purging and also address comorbid depression or anxiety.

Medication. The only FDA-approved medication for treating any eating disorder is fluoxetine (Prozac) for bulimia nervosa, at a dose of sixty milligrams per day.[30] The use of fluoxetine is associated with reductions in the core bulimia symptoms of binge eating and purging, as well as associated psychological features in the short term. In clinical trials, the sixty-milligram dose outperformed lower doses and was associated with prevention of relapse at one year. Unfortunately, many primary care physicians, and even psychiatrists, underdose bulimia nervosa. They will explain their hesitation by the age or weight of the patient, but the most common dose that individuals come to us on is twenty milligrams, and it is no wonder that they are not responding. Treatment with fluoxetine does not lead to a long-term cure, however. In fact, the optimal duration of treatment, and the optimal approach to maintain treatment gains when treating with fluoxetine, have not been established. Although practitioners in the community commonly prescribe Wellbutrin (bupropion) to patients with bulimia nervosa off-label, it has been known to cause seizures in individuals with eating disorders and is contraindicated in their care by the manufacturer.

Treatment for Binge Eating Disorder
Goals of Inpatient, Residential, Partial Hospitalization, and Outpatient Treatment. BED rarely requires inpatient hospitalization with the exception of medical stabilization. A few residential programs have emerged in recent years. Some of these programs have risen out of residential weight-loss programs that have realized that not addressing binge eating can seriously compromise weight-loss outcomes. These programs focus on dual outcomes of weight loss and abstinence from binge eating. Other programs eschew weight-loss goals and focus solely on abstinence from binge eating. As with bulimia nervosa, the vast majority of care for BED occurs in the outpatient setting. As noted earlier, self-help is viewed as the initial treatment of choice for BED in the United Kingdom, and a variety of books, computer programs, and smartphone apps are available to assist individuals with guiding their own treatment. Individual or group psychotherapy and medication management are the next most common approach, with the primary

treatment goal being abstinence from binge eating. Many treatments also focus on appetite awareness and incorporate weight control strategies into the intervention. Controversy exists, however, about whether weight loss should be a treatment goal for BED, as many patients claim that repeated attempts at weight loss were actually causal factors in their eating disorder and that healthy lifestyle regardless of weight loss is a more appropriate therapeutic goal (see box on page 283).

Psychotherapy. Self-help can be a valuable tool in the treatment of BED. Clinical trials looking at self-help treatment revealed decreases in binge eating as well as psychological features of BED. Self-help worked better than just putting patients on a waiting list for face-to-face treatment, at least in the short term, and abstinence rates were comparable to those seen in face-to-face treatment.

In examining psychotherapies for treating BED, CBT has been the most widely studied,[31] though there have been investigations of other treatments, including IPT, MI, and structured behavioral weight loss (BWL). BWL typically focuses on making changes to one's diet and physical activity to achieve weight loss. Both CBT and IPT are effective in reducing the frequency of binge eating, and CBT can help a significant number of patients achieve abstinence from binge eating. Adding an MI approach to psychotherapy also appears to boost results. CBT is effective in individual, group, and even guided-self-help approaches. All of these psychotherapies bring with them positive changes in psychological measures such as cognitive restraint, disinhibition, hunger, and shape and weight concerns.

The types of CBT that have been tested thus far do not reliably lead to weight loss. The reasons why weight gain is not a guaranteed outcome of abstinence from binge eating can be illustrated with simple math. Denise Wilfley, Ph.D., professor of psychiatry, medicine, pediatrics, and psychology at Washington University in St. Louis, presented a lucid description of why successful treatment of BED might not lead to weight loss. For her example, she chose a thirty-seven-year-old woman with a BMI of 35.7 kg/m² (5'7" and 228 pounds). Her calculated energy requirement for weight maintenance was 2,400 calories per day, which totals 72,000 calories per month. Examining her caloric intake while actively binge eating, she consumed on average 3,400 calories on binge days (four times per month) and 2,450 calories on nonbinge days (twenty-six days per month). Her total monthly caloric consumption with binges was [(4 × 3,400) + (26 × 2,450)] or 77,300 calories, which is 5,300 calories in excess of her caloric requirements or the equivalent of 2.65 pounds per month (a weight gain trajectory). By eliminating her binges (and eating her typical 2,450 calories per day) she eliminated 4 × (3,400 − 2,450) = 3,800 calories per month from her intake. After she achieved abstinence from binge eating, her monthly total consumption was then (2,450 × 30) or 73,500 calories, which is still 1,500 calories in excess of her caloric needs to maintain (not lose!) weight. So this simple math illustrates why eliminating binge eating alone does not necessarily lead to weight loss. Specialized approaches, including appetite awareness training (AAT),[32] BWL,[33] and appetite-focused cognitive behavioral therapy (CBT-A),[34] have been developed and tested in the treatment of BED, which may assist with addressing both binge eating and weight management. The most important goals of psychotherapy for BED are eliminating binge eating and restoring healthy eating and activity behaviors.

Medications. A wide range of medications have been tested in the treatment of BED, including classes of antidepressants (such as SSRIs, a combined serotonin, dopamine, and norepinephrine uptake inhibitor, and tricyclic antidepressants), an anticonvulsant, and appetite suppressants. In placebo-controlled studies, a high-dose SSRI (escitalopram, brand name Lexapro), two anticonvulsant medications (zonisamide and topiramate, brand names Zonegran and Topamax), a stimulant medication (atomoxetine, brand name Strattera), and an appetite suppressant (sibutramine, brand name Meridia) were all associated with significant decreases in binge eating frequency, weight, and BMI in overweight or obese patients with BED.[35] In contrast, in an open-label trial, memantine (brand name Namenda), a commonly prescribed Alzheimer's medication, did lead to decreases in binge eating but no change in weight. However, lamotrigine (Lamictal), an anticonvulsant, did not lead to decreases in binge eating or weight, but did show some promise in reducing metabolic parameters, such as glucose and triglyceride levels, commonly associated with obesity and the development of Type 2 diabetes. Given the comorbidity among BED, obesity, and Type 2 diabetes, the use of lamotrigine as an augmentation strategy in the treatment of obese individuals with BED is definitely worth further study. Although not specifically mentioned in the contraindications because BED is not an official diagnosis in DSM-IV, as we saw with bulimia nervosa, Wellbutrin (bupropion) may also cause seizures in individuals with BED and should not be routinely prescribed in its treatment.

One major shortcoming of the literature is that we do not have long-term follow-up data after drug discontinuation. Therefore, we simply do not know how long any observed changes in binge eating, depression, and weight persist.

Medication Plus Psychotherapy. In community practice, patients are often treated with a combination of psychotherapy and medication. Collectively, research suggests that combining medication and CBT may improve both binge eating and weight loss outcomes.

Follow-Up and Booster Sessions
Once you have completed a course of therapy, and you and your therapist have agreed that it is time to discontinue treatment,

have an open discussion about follow-up. Although some people like to make a clean break from therapy, others find that preprogrammed or ad hoc booster sessions are a valuable approach to preventing slips or relapses. Convincing insurance companies of this is not always as easy, but if you can handle it financially, and think it might be a good idea for you, then consider this with your therapist. A check-in after six months or a year, or a discussion about how and when to reinitiate treatment, may be valuable tools in your recovery toolbox. If you restart therapy in the future, it may not be as long as your initial course—you may just need a few sessions to plot the next segment of your recovery course—but it is a lot easier doing that with a therapist who knows you well than starting with someone new.

A HUSBAND'S WORDS

My name is Tommy, and I am married to a very courageous woman who has suffered from an eating disorder for the past five years. I have worked in the medical field as a paramedic and a nurse for more than twenty years. I met Margie at a hospital while working as a paramedic, we started dating, and we have been together for nineteen years. I never saw signs of mental illness. Margie is a person who is intelligent, witty, honest, and, to me, the most beautiful person in the world. Like most women I have known, Margie has always been concerned about her weight. To me, this was something that was not so unusual; on the contrary, I viewed it as her trying to live a healthy lifestyle.

Five years ago, after a surgical procedure, Margie started losing weight. Many people complimented her on her looks and asked her for her diet and exercise tips. I never gave any of this a moment's thought because I was proud of her. She was losing weight and accomplishing a goal she set out to do. I did not realize the extent of her disorder until she started having other health problems, such as syncopal episodes (passing out) and tachycardia (rapid heart rate). It was reported to me by her employer (a doctor) that he believed her to have an eating disorder. He pointed out the evidence: overexercising, skipping meals, and purging. Needless to say, this came as a shock to me. I was angry with myself for not picking up on the signs, and also angry because I felt betrayed. Margie was sent to a residential treatment facility, and received continued treatment at the Eating Disorders Program at the University of North Carolina at Chapel Hill. During her treatment, I was very happy that she was receiving the best care possible to combat this disease; however, I also felt anger and betrayal because I felt left out of the treatment process.

Everyone agrees that all family should be involved in the treatment; however, it is easier for the family to be involved if the patient is a minor. Once you reach age eighteen, then things become different. Under the Health Insurance Portability and Accountability Act (HIPAA) a person's treatment plan is protected as private information. Spouses cannot receive any information on how to help with any disease much less an eating disorder without the patient's permission. An eating disorder for adults is something that is private and something that the patient protects at all costs. They protect and covet the control they are experiencing and are steadfast in refusing to relinquish one ounce of the control that they have over their body. In our case, cooking, grocery shopping, clothes shopping, dealing with some activities of daily living are all triggers for Margie. I found this out only after we started doing couple therapy. Couple therapy about the eating disorder saved our marriage. Before, I was angry at Margie's therapists and doctors because she would reveal her fears to them and leave me out of the loop. In our couple therapy, UCAN (Uniting Couples in the treatment of Anorexia Nervosa), I learned to separate the disease process from Margie. I would encourage all husbands and significant others to do the same. This type of therapy can have a major impact on your lives and recovery.

I would like to say how proud I am of Margie. It takes a remarkable amount of courage to stand before the world saying this is who I am, where I have been, and where I am now in recovery. I am so proud of you. You will always be my girl.

—Tommy

Excerpted from www.unchealthcare.org/site/newsroom_OLD/news/2009/February/ucan?searchterm=nih.

AWARENESS AND ACTION

Sometimes the hardest place to start is getting on the Internet or picking up the phone to find out what treatment resources are available near you. It can also be a daunting task to sort through the hype and marketing to determine what types of services are available and who is delivering them. If you Google "eating disorders treatment" and the name of your state, you will invariably access a number of national paid advertisements, but digging deeper down the unpaid list will put you on the trail of resources available near you. There is no question that the density of hits is going to differ between, say, California and Wyoming, but it's a start.

Use this chapter to help you develop a list of questions you want to ask. What type of therapy is provided? What is the philosophy of the program/therapist? What type of training/

experience do the providers have? Do they use a multidisciplinary approach? What kind of insurance do they take? Be a wise consumer of health care. If possible, enlist someone else's help to assist you with sorting through all of the information. It is your life and your money; be as careful and thoughtful as you would be when buying a new house. You might be there for a while, and you want to make sure the foundation is sound and that it's a good fit.

CHAPTER 12

It's Not a Life Sentence, and Recovery Is Not Solitary Confinement

Frances, age thirty-seven, arrived in my office after having been "fired" by her previous psychologist. She settled immediately into the comfortable chair, folded up her legs, and wrapped her arms around them, as so many individuals with anorexia nervosa do. Her first words to me were, "I'm a lifer." She had first developed anorexia nervosa at age fifteen when she had high hopes of becoming a professional dancer. Her initial five years with the disorder were horrendous, with multiple hospitalizations, frequent visits to the emergency room, depression, anxiety, self-harm, and laxative, diuretic, and stimulant abuse that eventually generalized to alcohol and other drugs. Frances had eaten her way through treatment programs across the country, only to lose weight immediately after being discharged, starting the cycle all over. One therapist had labeled her a "lifer," which she adopted in her own self-description. When I asked her what she meant, she explained that 25 percent of people with anorexia nervosa are hopeless cases—and she was one of them.

Talk about starting therapy out with some negative expectations! As Frances's treatment unfolded, it became clear that her MO had become reducing therapists' expectations early and often. So many had given up on her in the past that she thought if she gave up on herself first, she could not be disappointed by their lack of belief in her ability to recover.

Somewhat strikingly, Frances had virtually lived a double life from ages twenty to thirty-seven, which is when she showed up in my office. She was married, had two children, drove them to soccer and dance practice, and helped them with their homework. Privately, however, she was trapped in perpetual anorexia hell. Frances's self-loathing manifested in ongoing starvation, occasional self-harm, and hair pulling, all of which occurred after her regular work and parenting duties. Her only emotional regulation tools physically damaged her body. Her husband traveled often, which opened the door for more self-destructive behaviors. In her daily life, Frances was accomplished and a supportive and loving mother who fiercely defended her pups. She had segregated her eating disorder outside of normal work and family hours, where it flourished and haunted her.

Frances had bought the line about being a "lifer" and resisted my encouragement to open up a discussion about the possibility of recovery. No doubt the thought of raising expectations again only to be fired by another therapist was simply too painful to consider. But gradually she started listening as we discussed all of the remarkable traits she possessed that allowed her to be such a wonderful mom and be a success at work—despite her ongoing pain. That those traits could be channeled toward recovery had not been in Frances's consciousness. We went very slowly down the path, not focusing on total recovery at first, but rather on more minor reprieves from her disordered eating and self-harm behaviors. Each small success chipped away at her "lifer" identity and opened the door ever so slightly to the possibility that this may not be a life sentence.

Frances experienced a few major setbacks, which were presented to me with an "I told you so" attitude, fully expecting me to either abandon her or give up on my efforts to work with her to reduce her symptoms. But, fully aware that recovery is never linear, I just held the reins for her until she could get back up on the horse. Frances realized then that I wasn't going anywhere, and that she had probably also met her match when it came to stubbornness and determination. Remaining calm during setbacks is probably the biggest gift that providers can give to their patients: Assessing danger, getting appropriate care, and hanging in there with them goes a long way toward building trust.

Frances reversed her "lifer" status and is no longer living a double life. Although no longer in treatment, she still occasionally checks in. At various points along the way, especially when major stresses loom, she feels the pull toward restriction. Even though she has developed effective and nonharmful emotional regulation skills (she started taking adult dance classes and rediscovered the joy she had experienced with dance), occasionally she'd find herself cutting back on food or pulling at her eyebrows unconsciously while driving. Frances developed enough self-awareness that she could view these tendencies as red flags for action rather than indices of failure. She would take stock and address the stressors directly in order to prevent slipping back into unhealthy behavior patterns. Frances's midlife pardon may have saved her from a lifelong self-fulfilling prophecy and possibly an even worse outcome.

Rebecka Peebles, M.D., an adolescent medicine physician and director of the Eating Disorders Program at the Children's Hospital of Philadelphia, has wise words to say about individuals with eating disorders across the life span, even though her practice caters primarily to children and adolescents. When asked at what point she draws the line and gives up hope, she states with conviction that for her, "There is no line." She says that everyone deserves the right to recover, and she acknowledges that recovery can happen at any time.

To think about recovery, it is helpful to consider three dimensions of functioning: physical, behavioral, and psychological.[1] Physical recovery generally refers to biological dimensions such as BMI, menstrual function, and medical complications. Behavioral recovery refers to the absence of any of the hallmark behaviors associated with eating disorders, such as fasting, restricting, binge eating, purging, and excessive exercising. Finally, psychological recovery refers to the psychological characteristics of eating disorders, such as the drive for thinness and body dissatisfaction, being within the healthy, "normal" range. Some believe that individuals who have physical and behavioral recovery, but not psychological recovery, should be referred to as remitted but not recovered. Although the amount of time an individual needs to be free of these symptoms to be considered recovered has not been codified, most practitioners would agree that a full year is a wise threshold to consider. We will review these three parameters for anorexia nervosa, bulimia nervosa, and BED and provide examples of recovered and not yet recovered individuals.

Remission, In Recovery, Recovered . . . a Rose by
Any Other Name
Our language to describe the course of recovery from eating disorders is wholly inadequate. Even among professionals, we can't agree what it means to be in remission, to relapse, or even whether complete recovery from an eating disorder is possible. Efforts are under way to develop a shared vocabulary and concrete definitions of these terms, but in the interim, it is most helpful to discuss conceptually what it means to be well, the definition of which may differ somewhat across the eating disorders. But before we go into specific examples, let's wrestle with the language.

People vary in whether they prefer to consider themselves to be "in recovery" versus "recovered." In part, this may be due to their conceptualization of their disorder and what motivates them to stay well. Individuals who have adopted a personal understanding of their eating disorder as being like an addiction may prefer to call themselves "in recovery." This model reflects the addiction field's belief that "once an addict, always an addict," and underscores the importance of abstinence from substances (or, in the case of eating disorders, from high-risk behaviors or foods) that could trigger a relapse. For many, viewing themselves as "in recovery" can be a motivator and a reminder that they remain vulnerable to relapse. However, some question whether this label may underestimate a person's ability to truly recover from an eating disorder. For example, if they always believe they are "in recovery," does that ever allow them to truly put the disorder behind them? I would argue that if viewing recovery as a journey is helpful in remaining well, then the "in recovery" label works well for them.

Others find it important to be able to reach a final stage of being "recovered" in order to state firmly that this stage of their life is behind them. Of course, being recovered does not mean that you are no longer at risk. One important fact is that, once you have had an eating disorder, you do remain at higher risk of another episode than someone who never had an eating disorder. The danger lies in believing that once recovered you are no longer vulnerable. Much like an ex-smoker who might occasionally get a whiff of a cigarette and think it might be awesome to have just one drag, someone with a history of anorexia nervosa might feel the same way about wanting to skip a meal, or to lose five pounds. Or someone who has recovered from bulimia nervosa might long for the release that just one purge might provide. Or someone with past BED might think wistfully about losing himself in just one binge on a particularly stressful day.

So, rather than argue about optimal terminology, perhaps the best solution is to see which fits best with you. If viewing your recovery as an ongoing journey suits you better, and if being "in recovery" helps you to be more mindful of traps or setbacks you might encounter, then by all means, call yourself "in recovery." In contrast, if the addiction model does you no favors, and it is important for you to definitively wrap up a particular phase of your life in order to move on, then be "recovered." Just remain mindful of that Achilles' heel and don't be lured into believing that you are invulnerable to future risk.

At the root of the recovery question is the extent to which symptoms continue to interfere with life. If symptoms are still distressing, or if they are interfering with your quality of life, then you have not yet reached the final stages of recovery.

Chronic Eating Disorders
Although one never gives up hope, chronic eating disorders do occur, and a subgroup of individuals live out their life with either smoldering symptoms or a pattern of waxing and waning that never seems to give way to sustained recovery. For this group of individuals, although recovery should never be entirely ruled out, more realistic goals may be optimizing quality of life, and minimizing periods of severe relapse requiring hospitalization.

Developing a rational follow-up plan in conjunction with your treatment team and support people, be they family or a partner or other caring individual, is the best way to avoid serious setbacks. With contingencies in place for alerting the treatment team when relapses are occurring, and clear plans for when hospitalization is indicated, tussles over procrastination or denial can be avoided. Individuals with chronic anorexia nervosa are able to collaborate with their team and loved ones more when they are doing relatively well. Thus, making these decisions when in the throes of a relapse is much more challenging, as thinking becomes more rigid, and denial and hopelessness can cloud decision making. If a plan is developed and agreed upon during a healthier period, it can serve as a road map for action when relapse occurs.

Chronic bulimia nervosa, purging disorder, and BED also

occur, and to some extent, the same principles apply. With bulimia and purging disorder, although prolonged hospitalization is less likely, a reasonable goal is to work toward a maintenance plan that reduces the number of emergency room visits due to dehydration, electrolyte imbalances, or other problems secondary to purging and dysregulated eating. Developing clear warning signs and a strategy that the treatment and support teams can implement when behavior is worsening is critical to early action and intervention. We know much less about chronic BED, although we do know that, for many, intermittent binge eating remains a lifelong pattern. As with all eating disorders, a focus on health parameters is paramount. In the case of BED, if the sufferer is also dealing with medical comorbidities associated with obesity, then ongoing monitoring of blood pressure, cholesterol, and other systems that can be affected by overweight can assist with monitoring the health aspects of BED.

For all eating disorders, readiness to change remains an important factor across the life span, and trying out a treatment that did not succeed in the past can be worthwhile. Even if someone did not benefit from CBT in their twenties, for example, that does not mean it is not worth trying again in their forties. Many people find that a second or even third go-around, years after their initial therapy, somehow takes hold in ways that the initial treatment did not. Perhaps it is therapist fit, or perhaps it is readiness to change on the part of the patient—or some critical combination of both—but giving treatment another go is always worth considering in the later stages of what appears to be a chronic illness.

IS THERE A ROLE FOR PALLIATIVE CARE IN ANOREXIA NERVOSA?

No topic evokes more emotion and controversy than the role of palliative care in cases of anorexia nervosa that are truly refractory to treatment. Although palliative care is commonly discussed with other diseases, there has been very little discourse about whether there should be a role for it in the management of anorexia nervosa, and, if yes, how and when it should be decided. That the topic stirs up so much emotion is testimony to the deeply held belief that we all feel that people should not die from this disorder. Yet out of respect for patients who have faced this decision, I include the topic in this book. I will start with a quote from Allan Kaplan, M.D., M.Sc., FRCP(C), chief of clinical research and director of research training at the Centre for Addiction and Mental Health in Toronto, Ontario, Canada, who underscores that palliative care does not mean giving up on a patient.

Palliative care focuses on providing patients with relief from the symptoms, pain, and stress of a serious illness—whatever the diagnosis and prognosis. The goal is to improve quality of life for both the patient and the family. The transition from aggressive to palliative care is often considered in the face of what is termed "medical futility," which is defined as "a clinical action serving no useful purpose in attaining a specified goal for a given patient." Futility itself means that a treatment cannot have the intended effect or that recovery is deemed impossible or highly unlikely. Although this term may have concrete and interpretable meaning with diseases such as terminal cancer, it is extremely complex when applied to anorexia nervosa.

Amy Lopez et al.[3] raise the possibility that palliative care may play a role in the care of treatment refractory anorexia nervosa when the patient is no longer responsive to treatment, when the patient continues to decline physiologically and psychologically, and when the patient faces an "inexorably terminal course." Unfortunately, we have no agreed-upon definition of treatment refractory anorexia nervosa, and patients with the disorder are often unresponsive to treatment, further highlighting the nuances of considering when palliative care is appropriate with this disorder.

Dr. Kaplan works with a community-based treatment model in which providers visit patients in a variety of settings (e.g., hospitals, hospice, group homes, personal, or family homes). The team's goals are social connection, quality of life, medical stability, and keeping patients out of the hospital. Patients enrolled in the program have high levels of chronicity and recidivism and often have compounding medical problems.

The decision to transition to palliative care is not an easy one. Kaplan underscores the importance of communication between the eating disorders team and the palliative care team, the inclusion of lawyers and bioethicists in decision making, and the inclusion of the patient and family at every decision point along the way of developing a palliative care plan. Common characteristics of patients he has transitioned to palliative care include: ill for more than fifteen years; through multiple hospitalizations without a sustained response; extensive nasogastric or jejunostomy tube refeeding; strongly requested that they no longer want to be hospitalized; understand the ramifications of their decision; have strong family support; and the family is in agreement with the decision. He does not view the transition to palliative care as giving up on recovery, but rather as a final chance for the patient to choose recovery or not. If the patient is involved in all decisions about care, it leaves the door to recovery open until the very end.

A palliative care approach in anorexia nervosa may mean no further involuntary treatment, no weigh-ins or caloric prescriptions, or no mandated psychotherapy. The components of palliative care are the same as for any terminal illness: 1) make sure the patient is comfortable and pain free; 2) make sure that the patient's basic needs are met for hygiene and bed care; 3) provide support and education for the patient and the parents; 4) explain to them exactly how the process of dying will unfold; 5) have the team be on call twenty-four hours a day so that the family/patient can reach out to them at any time.

Families may differ in what they seek from palliative care. For some, the struggle has become too overwhelming and they may opt for care outside the home with placement in a group home or hospice. Others could choose to have quiet family bonding time at home in contrast to chaotic years of living in hospitals. The transition to palliative care requires a paradigmatic shift in all involved. In many cases the patient wants to live, but does not want to—or is unable to—give up the disease. Or the patient remains in strict denial that she or he is in danger of dying. The shift enables the team to discuss how the patient can live with the disease, with improved quality of life, until the end comes or until a shift in attitudes toward recovery emerges.

A transition to palliative care may be welcome for the patient who can no longer tolerate the vigor of aggressive treatment. Patients who have been through multiple courses of refeeding and subsequent deterioration, who have been committed to treatment involuntarily, and who may have undergone multiple interventions that have failed, may opt for the comfort of palliative care over what has become the torture of ongoing interventions that they experience as medically futile. Of course, the question always looms whether an individual in such a compromised physical and mental state is competent to make a decision in favor of palliative care, which is precisely why the decision should always be made in conjunction with families, eating disorders providers, palliative care providers, lawyers, and bioethicists.

The concept of palliative care in anorexia nervosa is emotionally charged, but that is no reason to shy away from discussions. Many of us have seen instances of patients who we were sure were going to succumb to the disorder seemingly miraculously recover and go on to live rich lives. Regrettably, we have also seen individuals whose bodies have simply surrendered to the burden of the illness. Dr. Kaplan underscores that palliative care is not "giving up." He quotes a mother who explains, "It is the opposite of giving up; it provided us with a framework of treatment that met my daughter's needs and allowed her to spend her last period of her life comfortably, with dignity and surrounded by those who loved her." Whether the option of palliative care should be a component of our palette of interventions should remain an active area of discussion. It is a topic that clearly has important medical, legal, philosophical, spiritual, and ethical implications.

The Faces of Recovery

In order to paint a more human picture of what remission and recovery mean, here are some case examples that illustrate various degrees of wellness after suffering from the acute illness. Contrast the recovery and remission profiles to understand varying degrees with which ongoing symptoms can continue to influence quality of life for individuals in midlife with eating disorders.

Recovery from Anorexia Nervosa. Starting with anorexia nervosa, physical recovery is anchored in no longer being in the underweight category (BMI <18.5). Resumption of

menstruation for women is another indicator of physical recovery, as is the absence of other medical complications from
the disorder. Behavioral recovery means no restrictive eating,
fasting, binge eating, or compensatory behaviors, such as excessive exercise. I would suggest that another dimension of
behavioral recovery would include eating a wide variety of
foods from all food groups and not displaying food avoidance.
Psychological recovery is usually the last to emerge and includes having characteristics such as drive for thinness (or, for
some men, drive for muscularity or low body fat), fear of weight
gain, distorted body size perception, restraint, and weight and
shape concerns within the range of otherwise healthy individuals in the community. Rarely considered are all of the ancillary
symptoms that are not part of the diagnostic criteria for anorexia nervosa, such as body dissatisfaction, being able to eat
without anxiety, body checking, and restricted food choices.
These become difficult to pin down because they are repre-
sented to a large extent on a continuum in the community: At
what point does someone with a history of anorexia nervosa
approach the "normative discontent" of other women in the
community who are also dissatisfied with their bodies and
avoid certain foods? It is much harder to make these subtle
distinctions.

> * *Remitted from anorexia nervosa.* Paulina spent two
> months in a residential treatment program for anorexia
> nervosa and was discharged when she reached 90 per-
> cent of her ideal body weight, which was the equivalent
> of a BMI of 18.9. She had stopped purging when she was
> in the hospital and did not resume when she was back
> home. Before her hospitalization, Paulina would run for
> hours on the treadmill each day. Her husband had
> basically given her an ultimatum: the treadmill had to
> go or he would. She managed to keep her urges to
> exercise under control, which was somewhat easier after

she developed excruciating plantar fasciitis. Paulina kept her BMI at 18.9 to 19.0, but when she was at 19.0, she would become increasingly anxious. She still hated what she saw in the mirror and did rigid calorie math to make sure she was not eating any more than she was expending. *Paulina displayed physical and behavioral recovery, but not psychological recovery.*

* *Recovered from anorexia nervosa.* Estella was fourteen when she was first hospitalized for anorexia nervosa, and her BMI hovered around 18 for twenty years. After the loss of a child, she suffered a severe relapse and was rehospitalized at age thirty-four when her BMI reached 14. Estella completed inpatient treatment and partial hospitalization before being discharged to an excellent outpatient treatment team, with whom she worked intensively for four years. Both her husband and her daughter were included in treatment. Estella found motivation to recover in her daughter and in her faith. She struggled at first to keep weight on, still harboring a belief that she was responsible for her baby's death and thinking that she was not worthy of nourishment. But through family therapy and work with her church, she gradually transformed her thinking and began to accept her right to be happy and be engaged in the world. Her BMI went up to about 22, which would have sent her into a panic in the past, but she tolerated it as a sign of her choosing to live. Estella was binge, purge, and diet free for a year and felt truly liberated to no longer be plagued by constant thoughts about her body. Even when someone commented on her weight gain, she took it in stride and interpreted it as a sign that the person was glad that she was healthy. When she talked with her female friends, she swore she actually had more healthy attitudes about eating and weight than they did. She had replaced those body- and food-related thoughts with a

focus on her daughter, her family, her work, and her faith. *Estella achieved physical, behavioral, and psychological recovery.*

Recovery from Bulimia Nervosa. Physical recovery from bulimia nervosa generally means having laboratory values that are in the healthy range, having no episodes of dehydration, and having no other physical symptoms associated with bulimia nervosa. Behavioral recovery refers to the absence of both binge eating and purging behavior of any kind. Since the only psychological diagnostic criterion for bulimia nervosa is "undue influence of shape and weight on self-evaluation," psychological recovery would officially mean having a degree of shape and weight concern within the bounds of that displayed by otherwise healthy individuals. I would argue that true recovery would also include eating a wide variety of foods comfortably, without feeling urges to binge eat or purge, and developing healthy emotion regulation strategies that don't involve bulimic behaviors.

 * *Remitted from bulimia nervosa.* When he entered treatment, Luis was binge eating and self-inducing vomiting upward of five times a day. No one at work or home had any idea. His wife of ten years knew he had a tendency to "eat emotionally," and at one point, she had called him a "compulsive eater," but the true depths of his bulimia remained a secret even to her. Luis reluctantly joined a therapy group and developed many tools to reduce his binge eating and purging. He was proud of the changes he'd made, but he still struggled occasionally with social occasions. On Fridays after work, his creative team always went out for a drink, and they invariably got pizza, wings, or some other food that made him uncomfortable. Luis navigated most Fridays well by using the tools he learned in therapy, but every once in a while, he

just felt compelled to purge before going home. *Luis was on his way toward behavioral recovery, but he had not yet achieved complete abstinence from binge eating behaviors.*
* *Recovered from bulimia nervosa.* Hugh had been bulimic for a decade. He thought that, in order to attract a partner, he had to have the perfect body. He exercised, used supplements, dieted, and lifted every day—and then would binge and purge all weekend when his control gave way. When he met Peter and their relationship intensified, Hugh started to realize that Peter valued much more about him than his abs. Peter noticed that something was amiss with Hugh's eating and exercise behavior and confronted him with his concern. Peter even went to the doctor with him to get a treatment referral. Peter's sister had been bulimic, and he was keenly aware of the challenges of recovery. Hugh decided to put all of his energy into recovery and had an enormously supportive partner in Peter. He went for an entire year without binge eating or purging and learned how to enjoy exercising for health rather than driving himself into the ground in pursuit of physical perfection. *Hugh achieved physical, behavioral, and psychological recovery from bulimia nervosa.*

Recovery from Binge Eating Disorder Defining full recovery from BED poses an interesting challenge. If we use the same framework and look for physical, behavioral, and psychological recovery, we immediately face some dilemmas. First, what is physical recovery from BED? Does it include having a BMI in the healthy weight range? Although the casual observer might think so, this is an enormously controversial topic. The medical profession likes to look at two outcomes for BED treatment: abstinence from binge eating and weight regulation. Several groups of individuals are adamant about the fact that weight regulation should not be viewed as an outcome or a recovery criterion for BED. They contend that the fixation on weight loss and repeated attempts to lose weight over the years contributed to the disorder, and that using weight loss as an outcome only perpetuates that potential damaging focus (see box on page 283). If that's that case, then what are the physical symptoms of recovery from BED? For those who do have challenges with weight control, it could more meaningfully be having their blood pressure or cholesterol within healthy ranges, but these may be better defined as symptoms of obesity than symptoms of BED.

Behavioral symptoms are easier to define. Behavioral recovery from BED is sustained abstinence from binge eating. I would also add the ability to eat a wide and varied diet without distress or fear of loss of control over eating.

Psychological recovery is also a challenge to define based on DSM-5 criteria for binge eating disorder. If you look closely, there aren't really any psychological diagnostic criteria other than referring to how you feel after a binge (i.e., disgusted, depressed, or guilty) or that you are distressed about the presence of binge eating. There are no criteria such as those seen in anorexia or bulimia nervosa that hint at the underlying motivation for binge eating (e.g., self-evaluation is unduly influenced by body shape and weight). So if we stick to the diagnostic criteria, at this point we can only really define behavioral recovery from BED. I would propose that a true psychological recovery from BED means having an array of strategies to use to deal with emotions that have nothing to do with food.

> * *Remitted from BED.* Fiona started binge eating when she was pregnant with her second child. She had never had an eating disorder when she was younger, but she just developed such incredible cravings during the early part of her pregnancy. Then, when the cravings went away, she couldn't stop eating. Fiona knew she was gaining too

much weight, which couldn't be good for the baby, but she felt her eating was out of control. After the baby's birth, although her binges decreased in frequency, she still occasionally felt that same loss of control. *Fiona was on the path toward behavioral remission, but was not in recovery.*

* *Recovered from BED: Version 1.* Becky was a part-time receptionist in a physical therapist's office. Her hours had recently been reduced in a cost-saving move, which made it tight to cover her car and condo payments. As she had always done, Becky buried her worries in food. She bought food in bulk in attempt to save money, but then she would just end up eating it all. When she hit two hundred fifty pounds, Becky was desperate. She heard an advertisement for a clinical trial for BED on the radio and decided to reach out for treatment. After three months of CBT, she had her binge eating under control. At the year follow-up mark, she still had not binged, but her weight had not changed. She was about to try another diet to try to get the weight off, but she was afraid that it might trigger a relapse into bingeing. *Some would say that Becky is not recovered because her weight is still in the obese range. Let's look at an alternative view.*

* *Recovered from BED: Version 2.* When she hit two hundred fifty pounds, Becky was desperate. She heard an advertisement for a clinical trial for BED on the radio and decided to reach out for treatment. After three months of CBT, she had her binge eating under control. Becky's therapist urged her to focus more on health parameters— such as blood pressure and cholesterol levels, eating healthfully, and being active—and not to focus on the number on the scale. The therapist explained that the years of yo-yo dieting could have been a contributing factor to Becky's BED. At the year follow-up mark, Becky

still had not binged, and her weight had not changed, but her blood pressure was down to 120/77. Becky was able to come off of her statin medications for high cholesterol, was playing tennis weekly and lifting weights, and was eating a wide and varied diet. *Others would say that Becky is recovered because her binge eating is under control and, although she may still be overweight, she is fit and healthy.*

This controversy is likely to be played out in many arenas after the publication of DSM-5. Whether weight is viewed as an important outcome has widespread consequences. If insurance companies expect treatments to lead to both abstinence from binge eating and sustained weight loss, they might deny payment for interventions that lead to abstinence only. This would also be setting a higher bar for BED treatment than for other weight loss programs—with the exception of bariatric surgery, which does lead to considerable weight loss for the majority of patients.

THE HEALTH AT EVERY SIZE MOVEMENT

The Health at Every Size (HAES) movement is challenging the medical establishment's persistent focus on weight loss as necessary for achieving health. Linda Bacon, Ph.D., and Lucy Aphramor, R.D., the foremothers of the HAES movement, insist that adjusting your lifestyle habits with an eye toward improving markers of well-being, such as reduced blood pressure, lower cholesterol levels, reduced stress, increased energy, and improved self-esteem—independent of any weight loss at all—is a far more desirable goal for people of all sizes to pursue. They recommend that the health care community adopt an approach toward public health nutrition that "encourages individuals to concentrate on developing healthy habits rather than on weight management."

Some people have difficulty understanding the principles that the HAES movement stands for. For clarity, I asked Deb Burgard, Ph.D., a California psychologist, to frame recovery from BED in terms that are congruent with HAES principles. Her answer was thorough and enlightening.

Dr. Burgard takes issue with the focus of recovery being on weight loss and abstinence from binge eating. She states, "Real recovery depends on how the person is responding to their body cues, and how they are responding to the other aspects of life that got entangled with food (whatever they are for that unique individual)." Discussing weight, she explains, "Research continues to show that people of varying sizes can be healthy, and their health status depends largely on genetics and the health practices that they find sustainable to do within the context of their particular lives. Our interventions should be weight neutral—i.e., they should be agnostic about the weight a particular individual should be—and we should discover that weight by helping the person to live a healthy life and see what weight their body ends up being when they do that."

She takes her observations one step farther. "BED is partly an iatrogenic illness. It can in part be caused by the prescription of dieting—even in rats! The focus on weight loss, when we do not have interventions that provide lasting weight loss, is a terrible burden on patients and clinicians alike, and it unnecessarily complicates treatment. Everyone should be keeping their eyes on the prize, which is to regain the skill almost everyone is born with, to be able to seek food when hungry, and stop eating when satisfied."

Further, she delves into the meat of the HAES concerns with a focus on weight loss. "When people say they must prescribe weight loss because someone has a health condition that is correlated with higher weight, I think they forget that none of us has a way to safely and permanently change their weight. None of us has data showing that the health risks of a reduced-weight person are that of a never-fat person because there are not enough people who have maintained a stable low weight to find out. What we do have data for—abundant data over decades and decades—is that the pursuit of weight loss is almost always going to become weight cycling. Weight cycling is not benign, or a parallel to, say, trying and failing to stop smoking. When you are not smoking, your body is healing, but when you are suppressing your weight, you are turning on genes that will make food more palatable and metabolism more thrifty. Meanwhile, you are losing lean body mass, the engine of fuel consumption. Going through the weight cycle, you are making yourself fatter and possibly sicker; psychologically, you are making yourself feel out of control, ineffective, and deserving of the weight stigma you may experience. Some people are going to develop disordered eating or frank eating disorders as part of this process, including BED."

She then presents her solution. "All of this is completely unnecessary. We can all focus on the practices that help people become healthier, whether this results in weight change or not." Deb emphasizes, "What is under our control are the behavioral choices that fall within the range of what we find sustainable."

Finally, she makes a plea to call in the body police and make the playground safe for everyone. "I think if we are serious about health, rather than policing bodies, we will refocus our goals on making it possible for everyone, of any size or ability, to get enough recess. Recess, for me, stands for all the great opportunities to play, relax, and connect with people— and just have fun. And recess is no good at all if there is bullying on the playground. So weight stigma and the prescription of everyone having to be a predetermined weight is part of the problem making people sicker. We have to change this about our environments, along with having access to good food, being able to get restful sleep, having work that is satisfying, and being free from violence and harmful pollutants."

Hope, or Words of Wisdom from the Eyes of the Therapist
Through the course of my thirty years of treating eating disorders, I have watched thousands of individuals on their recovery journeys. My own clinical observations have led me to these ingredients to recovery.

* *Be patient and compassionate with yourself.* Treatment will not succeed if you are impatient. Eating disorders develop over time, and they go away over time. Patients who I have seen do well develop a kindness and patience toward themselves that absolves them from the tyranny of perfectionism. There is no perfect recovery.
* *Eat.* I am not being facetious. Whether you have anorexia nervosa, bulimia nervosa, purging disorder, BED, or some variation on the theme, eating is your friend and a critical key to recovery—especially if you do it regularly and in appropriate moderation. Not eating gets people with every conceivable eating disorder in trouble.
* *Expect bumps along the road.* Recovery is not linear. If you expect it to be linear, you will be disappointed. Sometimes it might feel like one step forward, two steps back. But don't just focus on the two steps back; remember the one step forward as well, and give yourself credit for it. It is like driving a car. While you are driving to your destiny (recovery), all sorts of obstacles might get thrown in your path. You might hit a pothole, get a flat tire, get stuck in traffic, but eventually (possibly with help from

others like a mechanic to help change a flat tire) you get yourself back on the road. Unexpected obstacles might make you switch lanes, slow down, or even pull over on the shoulder because you can't see in heavy rain—but you can always get yourself back on the road. Even a detour will eventually allow you to get back on track. Obstacles surely get thrown your way, but you get better at learning how to deal with them—because you learn from every obstacle and can respond in a more effective way the next time you encounter it.

* *Find something about yourself you can love.* The disconnect between what wonderful people my patients are and their abysmal self-esteem has been one of the most challenging and intriguing aspects of working with eating disorders. How can I, as a therapist, help these people see the wonderful things about them that I can see but that they cannot? How can I assure them that it is okay to feel good about some aspect of themselves? Patients who have done well have been able to lift their self-loathing sheath, if only a little, to recognize and come to love some aspect about themselves that they can view as positive. This is often the first foothold into developing the self-permission for recovery.

* *Be persistent.* Don't give up. If a round of treatment fails, do not become defeatist. Try something else, or try another round of the same thing. Eventually, after enough turning and tapping, the lid is going to come off the jar, and you'll be free to progress in recovery.

* *Practice radical honesty.* In many ways, I believe this is the most important key to recovery. Because of extreme anxiety and ambivalence about recovery, patients may often keep a few eating disorder secrets in their pockets. They participate 80 percent or maybe even 90 percent in therapy but withhold important details from me (and from their loved ones). I have seen a course of treatment

turn around when patients have given up this security blanket. Radical honesty can feel like jumping off the high dive blindfolded, but giving up all of the eating disorder secrets is an essential piece of recovery. I remember one patient saying, "You're going to figure it all out anyhow, so I may as well just tell you." This marked the beginning of "no secrets," and the turning point of her recovery.

* *Rely on your support team.* Recovery is difficult in a vacuum. Define your support team, whether it includes your therapist, physician, partner, parents, friends, or siblings. Be clear with them about what type of help you need and what role they are willing to play. Your sister who has two children under five might not want to be called in the middle of the night, but she may be more than willing to be there for you when the kids are in preschool. Know how they can help and when they can help, and reach out. It is their responsibility to tell you when they are not available—not yours to try and guess or mind read. Eating disorders prey on loneliness.

* *Pat yourself on the back, and accept it when others pat you on the back.* Don't let a treatment success fly by without acknowledgment. Recovery is hard work, and if you don't allow yourself to feel a sense of accomplishment when you make progress, it will not be a reinforcing experience. If you go for a week without binge eating, give yourself an "atta-girl" or "atta-boy." If your therapist compliments you on progress, take it, don't deflect it. Learn how to take a positive statement on board and how to give one to yourself.

* *Don't sit back and expect recovery to come knocking.* No one ever said that recovery was easy. Recovery is not for the meek. You need to go out and seek recovery and put muscle into achieving it. This means going to appointments when every single bone in your body is crying out

to stay in bed. This means being honest about a behavior you engaged in rather than carrying it around with you. This means fending off urges to engage in behavior that might be immediately gratifying but will hurt you in the long run. This means facing your fears full on, feeling the anxiety, and working through it. Some people mistakenly think that therapy is supposed to make you feel good. For a long portion of your therapy, you might leave each session feeling worse than when you walked in. This is natural. You're digging up some heavy stuff and working on some difficult topics and behaviors. As your recovery progresses, it is likely to feel less painful, and there may be more times when you feel better when you leave. But if you leave feeling good all the time, chances are good you aren't doing the hard work necessary to recover.

* *Don't hold on to a nugget.* This is related to practicing radical honesty, but it refers to holding on to one last vestige of the eating disorder—not wanting to add that last "feared food" to your diet, allowing yourself one purge per week, skipping breakfast on Sundays. In your mind, that nugget might just keep the lifeboat afloat in case you want to step back into the familiar eating disorder. But rather than being a lifeboat, it is a heavy anchor that will drag you back down to the bottom of the eating disorder sea. You have to let it all go and find healthier alternatives that allow you to achieve the same endpoint—be it security, control, calm, or whatever that nugget provides you with—in order to close the door on the eating disorder and move on to the next phase of your life.

On that note, I reiterate the wise words of Dr. Rebecka Peebles, who never gives up hope. Remission can happen; recovery can happen; quality of life can improve for those with a chronic illness. My journey is to continue to work toward greater understanding of these pernicious illnesses and to develop and improve treatments that will ease your recovery journey. Even in those darkest moments when recovery may seem elusive, keep your eye on the path. If you lose your way, ask for directions. We can't know in advance whether your recovery journey will be a brief and straightforward jaunt, a long and complicated odyssey, or something in between. Regardless of which it is, and regardless of whether your goal is recovery or improved quality of life, hope remains for a tomorrow that is better than today.

Acknowledgments

I am grateful to Lauren Janson and Susan Kleiman for their assistance with research and to Jennifer Claire Knight, Lauren Metzger, Susan Ngo, Allison Pfotzer, and India Harvey for fact-checking. Important insights from Cristin Runfola, Ph.D., Mark Warren, M.D., M.P.H., Millie Maxwell, Ph.D., and Tom Hildebrandt, Psy.D., helped enrich both the research and clinical material presented. I thank all of the individuals who have shared their personal stories and perspectives to help put a human face, heart, and soul to my discussion of these pernicious illnesses.

Resources

Academy for Eating Disorders (AED)
Located in Deerfield, Illinois, the Academy for Eating Disorders (AED) strives for both education and practicality as it grows along with the number of eating disorder cases it sees every year. Advocacy and understanding are the foundations of this well-respected academy.

AED is a global, multidisciplinary professional organization that provides cutting-edge professional training and education; inspires new developments in eating disorders research, prevention, and clinical treatments; and is the international source for state of the art information in the field of eating disorders.
www.aedweb.org
111 Deer Lake Road, Suite 100
Deerfield, IL 60015, USA
Telephone: (847) 498-4274
Fax: (847) 480-9282
E-mail: info@aedweb.org
On Facebook: Academy for Eating Disorders and Twitter @aedweb

Binge Eating Disorder Association (BEDA)
The Binge Eating Disorder Association (BEDA) was founded to help those who have BED, their friends and family, and those who treat the disorder. BEDA provides the individuals who suffer from BED the recognition and resources they deserve to begin a safe journey toward a healthy recovery. BEDA also

serves as a resource for providers of all kinds to prevent, diagnose, and treat the disorder. By establishing strong connections among members and sister organizations, BEDA's goal is to give everyone access to the tools they need to live with, treat, and, ultimately, prevent the disorder.
www.bedaonline.com
637 Emerson Place
Severna Park, MD 21146, USA
Telephone: (855) 855-BEDA (2332)
Fax: (410) 741-3037
E-mail: info@bedaonline.com
On Facebook: Binge Eating Disorder Association and Twitter @BEDAorg

Eating Disorders Coalition

The Eating Disorders Coalition's mission is "to advance the federal recognition of eating disorders as a public health priority." This is the group that lobbies on Capitol Hill in order to improve funding for research about, treatment of, and education on eating disorders. They also work toward better insurance coverage and the recognition of eating disorders as serious illnesses worthy of adequate insurance coverage.
www.eatingdisorderscoalition.org
720 7th Street NW, Suite 300
Washington, DC 20001, USA
Telephone: (202) 543-9570
On Facebook: Eating Disorders Coalition for Research, Policy & Action

Families Empowered and Supporting Treatment of Eating Disorders (F.E.A.S.T.)

F.E.A.S.T. is an international organization of and for parents and caregivers to help loved ones recover from eating disorders by providing information and mutual support, promoting evidence-based treatment, and advocating for research and education to reduce the suffering associated with eating disorders.
www.feast-ed.org/

P.O. Box 331
Warrenton, VA 20188, USA
Telephone: (540) 227-8518
Skype name: F.E.A.S.T.
E-mail: info@FEAST-ED.org
On Facebook: F.E.A.S.T. (Families Empowered And Supporting
Treatment of Eating Disorders) and Twitter @FEASTtweets

Health at Every Size (HAES)
HAES is based on the simple premise that the best way to
improve health is to honor your body. It supports people in
adopting health habits for the sake of health and well-being
(rather than weight control).
www.haescommunity.org

National Association for Males with Eating Disorders (N.A.M.E.D.)
N.A.M.E.D. provides support to and resources about men with
eating disorders.
www.NAMEDinc.org
Christopher Clark
Executive Director
N.A.M.E.D
118 Palm Dr. # 11
Naples, FL 34112, USA
Telephone: (877) 780-0080 toll-free or (239) 775-1145
E-mail: Chris@NAMEDinc.org
On Facebook: National Association for Males with Eating
Disorders

National Eating Disorders Association (NEDA)
The National Eating Disorders Association (NEDA) is the largest
not-for-profit organization in the United States working to prevent
eating disorders and provide treatment referrals to those suffering
from anorexia, bulimia, and BED and those concerned with body
image and weight issues. NEDA sponsors National Eating Disorders Awareness Week, which takes place every year in February.

www.nationaleatingdisorders.org
165 West 46th Street
New York, NY 10036, USA
Telephone: 1 (800) 931-2237 toll-free or (212) 575-6200
Fax: (212) 575-1650
E-mail: info@NationalEatingDisorders.org
On Facebook: National Eating Disorders Association and
Twitter @NEDAstaff

National Institute of Mental Health (NIMH)

Long recognized as a "go-to source" for all things mental health,
the National Institute of Mental Health (NIMH) offers a wide
variety of information and services for those in need. The
NIMH provides information to help people better understand
mental health, mental disorders, and behavioral problems.
NIMH does not provide referrals to mental health professionals
or treatment for mental health problems.
www.nimh.nih.gov
6001 Executive Boulevard
Room 8184, MSC 9663
Bethesda, MD 20892-9663, USA
Telephone: 1 (866) 615-6464 toll-free or (301) 443-4513
Fax: (301) 443-4279
E-mail: nimhinfo@nih.gov
On Facebook: National Institute of Mental Health and Twitter
@NIMHgov

The Rudd Center for Food Policy and Obesity

The Rudd Center for Food Policy and Obesity at Yale University
is a nonprofit research and public policy organization devoted to
improving the world's diet, preventing obesity, and reducing
weight stigma. Their resource-rich website includes reports,
newsletters, informational videos, and podcasts to help families
with all aspects of food and nutrition.
www.YaleRuddCenter.org
309 Edwards Street

New Haven, CT 06511, USA
Telephone: (203) 432-6700
Fax: (203) 432-9674
On Facebook: Yale Rudd Center and Twitter @YaleRuddCenter

Beating Eating Disorders (beat) (United Kingdom)
beat provides help lines, online support and a network of
UK-wide self-help groups to help adults and young people in the
United Kingdom beat their eating disorders.
www.b-eat.co.uk/
Wensum House
103 Prince of Wales Road
Norwich
Norfolk
NR1 1DW, United Kingdom
Telephone: +44 (0)300 123 3355
E-mail: info@b-eat.co.uk
On Facebook: beat and Twitter @beatED

The Butterfly Foundation (Australia)
The Butterfly Foundation is dedicated to bringing about change
to the culture, policy, and practice in the prevention, treatment,
and support of those affected by eating disorders and negative
body image.
www.thebutterflyfoundation.org.au
Victoria
P.O. Box 453
Malvern VIC 3144, Australia
Telephone: + 61(0)3 9822 5771
New South Wales
103 Alexander Street
Crows Nest NSW 2065, Australia
Telephone: +61 (0)2 9412 4499
info@thebutterflyfoundation.org.au
On Facebook: The Butterfly Foundation and Twitter
@Bfoundation

Eating Difficulties Education Network (EDEN) (Auckland, New Zealand)
EDEN is a nonprofit community agency based in Auckland, New Zealand. Their purpose is to promote body trust and satisfaction, size acceptance, and diversity on an individual and societal level.
www.eden.org.nz
395A Manukau Road
Epsom, Auckland, New Zealand
P.O. Box 26 713, Epsom 1023, Auckland, New Zealand
Telephone: +64 (0)9 378 9039
E-mail: info@eden.org.nz
On Facebook: Eden Auckland and Twitter @EDENAuckland

Eating Disorders Association of New Zealand (EDANZ)
EDANZ was established to provide support and education for parents and caregivers of people with eating disorders. The society was established in September 2007 by a group of Auckland parents who all have children with eating disorders.
www.ed.org.nz
Telephone: +64 (0)9 5222679
E-mail: info@ed.org.nz

National Eating Disorder Information Centre (NEDIC)
The National Eating Disorder Information Centre (NEDIC) is a Canadian nonprofit organization that provides information and resources on eating disorders and weight preoccupation. Their goal is to promote healthy lifestyles that allow people to be fully engaged in their lives.
http://www.nedic.ca
200 Elizabeth Street
Toronto, Ontario, Canada
Telephone: (866) NEDIC-20 (866-633-4220) toll-free or Toronto (416) 340-4156
On Facebook: NEDIC—National Eating Disorder Information Centre and Twitter @nedic85

Notes

CHAPTER 1: A CULTURE OF DISCONTENT: WHY MIDLIFE AND WHY NOW?

1   Andrew Adam Newman, "Orthodontists Market to Adults Seeking Prettier Smiles." *New York Times*, February 1, 2012.

2   "2010 Census," U.S. Census Bureau, 2010, Table 1, www.census .gov/prod/cen2010/briefs/c2010br-03.pdf.

CHAPTER 2: DEFINING THE DISORDERS: WHAT ARE THESE EATING AND FEEDING DISORDERS?

1   American Psychiatric Association, *Diagnostic and Statistical Manual of Mental Disorders (DSM-I)*. Washington, DC: American Psychiatric Association, 1952; *Diagnostic and Statistical Manual of Mental Disorders (DSM-II)*. Washington, DC: American Psychiatric Association, 1968; *Diagnostic and Statistical Manual of Mental Disorders. Third Edition*. Washington, DC: American Psychiatric Association Press, 1980; *Diagnostic and Statistical Manual of Mental Disorders. Edition III-R. Third Edition*, revised. Washington, DC: American Psychiatric Association Press, 1987; *Diagnostic and Statistical Manual for Psychiatric Disorders: Fourth Edition*. Washington, DC: American Psychiatric Association Press, 1994; "DSM-5 Development." http://www.dsm5.org/Pages/Default.aspx; and Rick Mayes and Allan V. Horwitz, "DSM-III and the Revolution in the Classification of Mental Illness." *Journal of the History of the Behavioral Sciences* 41, no. 3 (2005): 249–67.

2   Daniel Le Grange, Sonja Swanson, Scott Crow, and Kathleen Merikangas, "Eating Disorder Not Otherwise Specified

Presentation in the US Population." *International Journal of Eating Disorders* 45, no. 5 (2012): 711–8.

3   American Psychiatric Association, "K 06 Feeding or Eating Disorder Not Elsewhere Classified." http://www.dsm5.org/ProposedRevision/Pages/proposedrevision.aspx?rid=26.

4   "The Food F.A.D. Study (Finicky Eating in Adults)," http://www.dukehealth.org/clinicaltrials/the_food_fad_study_finicky_eating_in_adults.

5   James Hudson, Eva Hiripi, Harrison Pope Jr., and Ronald Kessler, "The Prevalence and Correlates of Eating Disorders in the National Comorbidity Survey Replication." *Biological Psychiatry* 61, no. 3 (2007): 348–58.

6   Ruth Striegel-Moore, Faith Dohm, Helena Kraemer, C. Barr Taylor, Stephen Daniels, Patricia Crawford, and George Schreiber, "Eating Disorders in White and Black Women." *American Journal of Psychiatry* 160, no. 7 (2003): 1326–31.

7   Johannes Hebebrand and Cynthia Bulik, "Critical Appraisal of the Provisional DSM-5 Criteria for Anorexia Nervosa and an Alternative Proposal." *International Journal of Eating Disorders* 44, no. 8 (2011): 665–78.

8   Andrea Poyastro Pinheiro, Laura Thornton, Katherine Plotonicov, Federica Tozzi, Kelly Klump, Wade Berrettini, Harry Brandt, Steven Crawford, Scott Crow, Manfred Fichter, David Goldman, Katherine Halmi, Craig Johnson, Allan Kaplan, Pamela Keel, Maria LaVia, James Mitchell, Alessandro Rotondo, Michael Strober, Janet Treasure, D. Blake Woodside, Ann Von Holle, Robert Hamer, Walter Kaye, and Cynthia Bulik, "Patterns of Menstrual Disturbance in Eating Disorders." *International Journal of Eating Disorders* 40, no. 5 (2007): 424–34.

9   Unna Danner, Nicole Sanders, Paul Smeets, Floor van Meer, Roger Adan, Hans Hoek, and Annamarie van Elburg, "Neuropsychological Weaknesses in Anorexia Nervosa: Set-Shifting, Central Coherence, and Decision Making in Currently Ill and Recovered Women." *International Journal of Eating Disorders* 45, no. 5 (2012): 685–94

10 D. Catherine Walker, Drew Anderson, and Thomas Hildebrandt, "Body Checking Behaviors in Men." *Body Image* 6, no. 3 (2009): 164–70.

11 National Health Service Information Centre, NatCen, and University of Leicester, "Adult Psychiatric Morbidity Survey,"

ed. Sally McManus, Howard Meltzer, Traolach Brugha, Paul Bebbington, and Rachel Jenkins, 2009; John F. Morgan, Fiona Reid, and J. Hubert Lacey. "The SCOFF Questionnaire: Assessment of a New Screening Tool for Eating Disorders." *British Medical Journal* 319, no. 7223 (1999): 1467–8.

12 Hudson et al., "The Prevalence and Correlates of Eating Disorders in the National Comorbidity Survey Replication."

13 Ibid.

14 Sara Trace, Laura Thornton, Tammy Root, Suzanne Mazzeo, Paul Lichtenstein, Nancy L. Pedersen, and Cynthia Bulik, "Effects of Reducing the Frequency and Duration Criteria for Binge Eating on Lifetime Prevalence of Bulimia Nervosa and Binge Eating Disorder: Implications for DSM-5." *International Journal of Eating Disorders* 45, no. 4 (2012): 531–6.

15 Pamela Keel, Alissa Haedt, and Crystal Edler, "Purging Disorder: An Ominous Variant of Bulimia Nervosa?" *International Journal of Eating Disorders* 38, no. 3 (2005): 191–9.

16 Pamela Keel, Barbara Wolfe, Julie Gravener, and David Jimerson, "Co-Morbidity and Disorder-Related Distress and Impairment in Purging Disorder." *Psychological Medicine* 38, no. 10 (2008): 1435–42.

17 Sanna Tholin, Anna Karin Lindroos, Per Tynelius, Torbjörn Akerstedt, Albert J. Stunkard, Cynthia Bulik, and Finn Rasmussen, "Prevalence of Night Eating in Obese and Non-obese Twins." *Obesity* 17, no. 5 (2009): 1050–5; Ruth Striegel-Moore, Debra Franko, Douglas Thompson, Sandra Affenito, Alexis May, and Helena Kraemer, "Exploring the Typology of Night Eating Syndrome." *International Journal of Eating Disorders* 41, no. 5 (2008): 411–8; Tammy Root, Laura Thornton, Anna Karin Lindroos, Albert J. Stunkard, Paul Lichtenstein, Nancy L. Pedersen, Finn Rasmussen, and Cynthia Bulik, "Shared and Unique Genetic and Environmental Influences on Binge Eating and Night Eating: A Swedish Twin Study." *Eating Behaviors* 11, no. 2 (2010): 92–8; and Martina de Zwaan, Deborah Roerig, Ross Crosby, Sammy Karaz, and James Mitchell, "Nighttime Eating: A Descriptive Study." *International Journal of Eating Disorders* 39, no. 3 (2006): 224–32.

18 Deborah Beidel, Cynthia Bulik, and Melinda Stanley, *Abnormal Psychology*. Second Edition. Upper Saddle River, NJ: Pearson Publishing, 2011.

CHAPTER 3: WHAT'S DIFFERENT ABOUT MIDLIFE EATING DISORDERS?

1　Phillipa Hay, Jonathan Mond, Petra Buttner, and Anita Darby, "Eating Disorder Behaviors Are Increasing: Findings from Two Sequential Community Surveys in South Australia." *PloS One* 3, no. 2 (2008): e1541.

2　Martin R. Yeomans, "Effects of Alcohol on Food and Energy Intake in Human Subjects: Evidence for Passive and Active Over-Consumption of Energy." *British Journal of Nutrition* 92 Suppl. 1 (2004): S31–4.

3　Cynthia Bulik and Ted Reichborn-Kjennerud, "Medical Morbidity in Binge Eating Disorder." *International Journal of Eating Disorders* 34 Suppl. (2003): S39–46.

4　Nuray Kanbur and Debra Katzman, "Physical Signs and Symptoms Associated with Eating Disorders." In *Restoring Our Bodies, Reclaiming Our Lives*, ed. Aimee Liu. Boston and London: Trumpeter, 2011.

5　James Mitchell, Sheila Specker, and Martina De Zwaan, "Comorbidity and Medical Complications of Bulimia Nervosa." *Journal of Clinical Psychiatry* 52 Suppl. (1991): 13–20.

6　Ruth Striegel, Richard Bedrosian, Chun Wang, and Steven Schwartz, "Why Men Should Be Included in Research on Binge Eating: Results from a Comparison of Psychosocial Impairment in Men and Women." *International Journal of Eating Disorders* 45, no. 2 (2012): 233–40.

7　Fernando Fernandez-Aranda, Andrea Pinheiro, Federica Tozzi, Laura Thornton, Manfred Fichter, Katherine Halmi, Allan Kaplan, Kelly Klump, Michael Strober, D. Blake Woodside, Scott Crow, James Mitchell, Alessandro Rotondo, Pamela Keel, Katherine Plotnicov, Wade Berrettini, Walter Kaye, Steven Crawford, Craig Johnson, Harry Brandt, Maria La Via, and Cynthia Bulik, "Symptom Profile of Major Depressive Disorder in Women with Eating Disorders." *Australian and New Zealand Journal of Psychiatry* 41, no. 1 (2007): 24–31.

8　Suzanne Mazzeo, Margarita Slof-Op't Landt, Ian Jones, Karen Mitchell, Kenneth Kendler, Michael Neale, Steven Aggen, and Cynthia Bulik, "Associations Among Postpartum Depression, Eating Disorders, and Perfectionism in a Population-Based Sample of Adult Women." *International Journal of Eating Disorders* 39, no. 3 (2006): 202–11.

9   Walter Kaye, Cynthia Bulik, Laura Thornton, Nichole
    Barbarich, Kim Masters, and Price Foundation Collaborative
    Group, "Comorbidity of Anxiety Disorders with Anorexia and
    Bulimia Nervosa." *American Journal of Psychiatry* 161 (2004):
    2215–21.

10 Thomas Raney, Laura Thornton, Wade Berrettini, Harry
    Brandt, Steven Crawford, Manfred Fichter, Katherine Halmi,
    Craig Johnson, Allan Kaplan, Maria LaVia, James Mitchell,
    Alessandro Rotondo, Michael Strober, D. Blake Woodside,
    Walter Kaye, and Cynthia Bulik, "Influence of Overanxious
    Disorder of Childhood on the Expression of Anorexia Nervosa."
    International Journal of Eating Disorders 41, no. 4 (2008):
    326–32.

11 Mae Lynn Reyes-Rodríguez, Ann Von Holle, Teresa Ulman,
    Laura Thornton, Kelly Klump, Harry Brandt, Steven Craw-
    ford, Manfred Fichter, Katherine Halmi, Thomas Huber,
    Craig Johnson, Ian Jones, Allan Kaplan, James Mitchell,
    Michael Strober, Janet Treasure, D. Blake Woodside, Wade
    Berrettini, Walter Kaye, and Cynthia Bulik, "Posttraumatic
    Stress Disorder in Anorexia Nervosa." *Psychosomatic Medicine*
    73, no. 6 (2011): 491–7; Nathalie Godart, Martine Flament,
    Fabienne Perdereau, and Philippe Jeammet, "Comorbidity
    Between Eating Disorders and Anxiety Disorders: A Review."
    International Journal of Eating Disorders 32, no. 2 (2002).
    253–70.

12 Takuya Sawaoka, Rachel Barnes, Kerstin Blomquist, Robin
    Masheb, and Carlos Grilo, "Social Anxiety and Self-
    Consciousness in Binge Eating Disorder: Associations with
    Eating Disorder Psychopathology." *Comprehensive Psychiatry*
    53, no. 6 (2012): 740–5.

13 Hans-Christoph Steinhausen, "The Outcome of Anorexia
    Nervosa in the 20th Century." *American Journal of Psychiatry*
    159, no. 8 (2002): 1284–93.

14 Hans-Christoph Steinhausen and Sandy Weber, "The Out-
    come of Bulimia Nervosa: Findings from One-Quarter
    Century of Research." *American Journal of Psychiatry* 166, no.
    12 (2009): 1331–41.

15 Manfred Fichter, Norman Quadflieg, and Anna Gnutzmann,
    "Binge Eating Disorder: Treatment Outcome over a 6-Year
    Course." *Journal of Psychosomatic Research* 44, no. 3–4 (1998):
    385–405.

16   Harrison Pope Jr., Justine Lalonde, Lindsay Pindyck, B.
      Timothy Walsh, Cynthia Bulik, Scott Crow, Susan McElroy,
      Norman Rosenthal, and James Hudson, "Binge Eating Disor-
      der: A Stable Syndrome." *American Journal of Psychiatry* 163,
      no. 12 (2006): 2181–3.

17   Patrick Sullivan, "Mortality in Anorexia Nervosa." *American
      Journal of Psychiatry* 152, no. 7 (1995): 1073–74.

18   C. Laird Birmingham, Jenny Su, Julia A. Hlynsky, Elliot
      Goldner, and Min Gao, "The Mortality Rate from Anorexia
      Nervosa." *International Journal of Eating Disorders* 38, no. 2
      (2005): 143–46.

19   E. Clare Harris and Brian Barraclough, "Excess Mortality
      of Mental Disorder." *British Journal of Psychiatry* 173 (1998):
      11–53.

20   Jon Arcelus, Alex J. Mitchell, Jakie Wales, and Søren Nielsen,
      "Mortality Rates in Patients with Anorexia Nervosa and Other
      Eating Disorders: A Meta-Analysis of 36 Studies." *Archives of
      General Psychiatry* 68, no. 7 (2011): 724–31.

21   Antonio Preti, Marco Rocchi, Davide Sisti, Maria Valeria
      Camboni, and Paola Miotto, "A Comprehensive Meta-Analysis
      of the Risk of Suicide in Eating Disorders." *Acta Psychiatrica
      Scandinavica* 124, no. 1 (2011): 6–17.

22   Cynthia Bulik, Laura Thornton, Cristin Runfola, Emily
      Pisetsky, Thomas Frisell, Paul Lichtenstein, and Andreas
      Birgegård, "Suicide and Eating Disorders" (in progress).

23   Janet Treasure, Tara Murphy, George Szmukler, Gill Todd,
      Kay Gavan, and J. Joyce, "The Experience of Caregiving for
      Severe Mental Illness: A Comparison Between Anorexia
      Nervosa and Psychosis." *Social Psychiatry and Psychiatric
      Epidemiology* 36, no. 7 (2001): 343–7.

24   Ronald Kessler and Richard Frank, "The Impact of Psychiatric
      Disorders on Work Loss Days." *Psychological Medicine* 27, no.
      4 (1997): 861–73.

25   Jonathan Mond, Bryan Rodgers, Phillipa Hay, Ailsa Korten,
      Cathy Owen, and Peter Beumont, "Disability Associated with
      Community Cases of Commonly Occurring Eating Disorders."
      Australian and New Zealand Journal of Public Health 28, no. 3
      (2004): 246–51.

26   *The Global Burden of Disease: 2004 update.* World Health
      Organization 2008, 2004.

27   Jonathan Mond and Phillipa Hay, "Functional Impairment

Associated with Bulimic Behaviors in a Community Sample of Men and Women." *International Journal of Eating Disorders* 40, no. 5 (2007): 391–8.

28   Mike Green, Nicola Elliman, Anthony Wakeling, and Peter Rogers, "Cognitive Functioning, Weight Change and Therapy in Anorexia Nervosa." *Journal of Psychiatric Research* 30, no. 5 (1996): 401–10.

29   David Moser, Michelle Benjamin, John Bayless, Bradley McDowell, Jane Paulsen, Wayne Bowers, Stephen Arndt, and Arnold Andersen, "Neuropsychological Functioning Pretreatment and Posttreatment in an Inpatient Eating Disorders Program." *International Journal of Eating Disorders* 33, no. 1 (2003): 64–70.

30   Myra Cooper and Christopher Fairburn, "Thoughts About Eating, Weight and Shape in Anorexia Nervosa and Bulimia Nervosa." *Behaviour Research and Therapy* 30, no. 5 (1992): 501–11.

31   Mike Green et al., "Cognitive Functioning, Weight Change and Therapy in Anorexia Nervosa."

32   Paolo Cavedini, Tommaso Bassi, Alessandro Ubbiali, Alessia Casolari, Silvia Giordani, Claudia Zorzi, and Laura Bellodi, "Neuropsychological Investigation of Decision-Making in Anorexia Nervosa." *Psychiatry Research* 127, no. 3 (2004): 259–66.

33   Michael Strober and Craig Johnson, "The Need for Complex Ideas in Anorexia Nervosa: Why Biology, Environment, and Psyche All Matter, Why Therapists Make Mistakes, and Why Clinical Benchmarks Are Needed for Managing Weight Correction." *International Journal of Eating Disorders* 45, no. 2 (2012): 155–78.

34   Lesley Alderman, "Treating Eating Disorders and Paying for It." *New York Times*, December 3, 2010; South Carolina Department of Mental Health. "Eating Disorder Statistics," http://www.state.sc.us/dmh/anorexia/statistics.htm.

35   Pro Bono Economics, "Costs of Eating Disorders in England: Economic Impacts of Anorexia Nervosa, Bulimia Nervosa and Other Disorders, Focussing on Young People." London: BEAT, 2012.

36   Alderman, "Treating Eating Disorders and Paying for It."

37   Scott Crow, Maria Frisch, Carol Peterson, Jillian Croll, Susan Raatz, and John Nyman, "Monetary Costs Associated with

Bulimia." *International Journal of Eating Disorders* 42, no. 1 (2009): 81–3.

38   National Eating Disorders Association, "Media Watchdog," http://www.nationaleatingdisorders.org/programs-events/media -watchdog.php.

39   Laura Stampler, "Yoplait Pulls Ad Said to Promote Eating Disorders," http://www.huffingtonpost.com/2011/06/15/yoplait -pulls-ad-that-pos_n_877618.html#s292650&title=iMac.

CHAPTER 4: THE FACE OF EATING DISORDERS IN MEN

1   Ruth Striegel-Moore, Francine Rosselli, Nancy Perrin, Lynn DeBar, G. Terrance Wilson, Alexis May, and Helena Kraemer, "Gender Difference in the Prevalence of Eating Disorder Symptoms." *International Journal of Eating Disorders* 42, no. 5 (2009): 471–4.

2   Mae Lynn Reyes-Rodríguez, Debra Franko, Anguelique Matos-Lamourt, Cynthia Bulik, Ann Von Holle, Luis Camara-Fuentes, Dianisa Rodriguez-Anglero, Sarah Cervantes-Lopez, and Alba Suarez-Torres, "Eating Disorder Symptomatology: Prevalence Among Latino College Freshmen Students." *Journal of Clinical Psychology* 66, no. 6 (2010): 666–79.

3   James Hudson, Eva Hiripi, Harrison Pope Jr., and Ronald Kessler, "The Prevalence and Correlates of Eating Disorders in the National Comorbidity Survey Replication." *Biological Psychiatry* 61, no. 3 (2007): 348–58.

4   National Health Service Information Centre, "Adult Psychiatric Morbidity Survey," 2009.

5   Phillipa Hay, Jonathan Mond, Petra Buttner, and Anita Darby, "Eating Disorder Behaviors Are Increasing: Findings from Two Sequential Community Surveys in South Australia." *PloS One* 3, no. 2 (2008): e1541.

6   Charles Anderson and Cynthia Bulik, "Gender Differences in Compensatory Behaviors, Weight and Shape Salience, and Drive for Thinness." *Eating Behaviors* 5, no. 1 (2004): 1–11.

7   Kaori Shoji, "In Japan, It's the Men Who Want to Be Skinny and Cute." *New York Times*, November 19, 2007.

8   Ruth Striegel, Richard Bedrosian, Chun Wang, and Steven Schwartz, "Why Men Should Be Included in Research on Binge Eating: Results from a Comparison of Psychosocial

Impairment in Men and Women." *International Journal of Eating Disorders* 45, no. 2 (2012): 233–40.

9   Michael Strober, Roberta Freeman, Carlyn Lampert, Jane Diamond, and Walter Kaye, "Males with Anorexia Nervosa: A Controlled Study of Eating Disorders in First-Degree Relatives." *International Journal of Eating Disorders* 29, no. 3 (2001): 263–9.

10 Ted Reichborn-Kjennerud, Cynthia Bulik, Kenneth Kendler, Hermine Maes, Espen Røysamb, Kristian Tambs, and Jennifer Harris, "Gender Differences in Binge-Eating: A Population-Based Twin Study." *Acta Psychiatrica Scandinavica* 108, no. 3 (2003): 196–202.

11 Jere Longman, "Battle of Weight Versus Gain in Ski Jumping." *New York Times*, February 11, 2010.

12 Ibid.

13 International Ski Federation. "Specifications for Competition Equipment Edition 2011/2012." 2011.

14 Will Graves and Jeff McMurray, "Jockeys Still Battle Weight Issues, but Progress Being Made," ESPN, http://sports.espn.go .com/espn/wire?section=horse&id=3367868.

15 Centers for Disease Control and Prevention. "Safety and Health in the Horse Racing Industry," ed. National Institute for Occupational Safety and Health (NIOSH), 2009.

16 Shaun Riehl, Andrew Subudhi, Jeffery Broker, Kim Schenck, and Jaqueline Berning, "The Prevalence of Subclinical Eating Disorders Among Male Cyclists." *Journal of the American Dietetic Association* 107, no. 7 (2007): 1214–7.

17 Catherine Pearson, "Male Athletes Struggle with Eating Disorders." Huffington Post, http://www.huffingtonpost.com /2011/08/16/eating-disorders-men_n_928206.html.

18 Antonia Baum, "Eating Disorders in the Male Athlete." *Sports Medicine* 36, no. 1 (2006): 1–6.

19 Arnold Andersen, Tureka Watson, and Janet Schlechte, "Osteoporosis and Osteopenia in Men with Eating Disorders." *Lancet* 355, no. 9219 (2000): 1967–8.

20 Philip Mehler, Allison Sabel, Tureka Watson, and Arnold Andersen, "High Risk of Osteoporosis in Male Patients with Eating Disorders." *International Journal of Eating Disorders* 41, no. 7 (2008): 666–72.

21 Søren Nielsen, Susanne Møller-Madsen, Torben Isager, Jan Jorgensen, Katrine Pagsberg, and Sten Theander, "Standardized

Mortality in Eating Disorders: A Quantitative Summary of Previously Published and New Evidence." *Journal of Psychosomatic Research* 44, no. 3–4 (1998): 413–34.

22   Ted Reichborn-Kjennerud et al., "Gender Differences in Binge-Eating: A Population-Based Twin Study."

23   Thomas Joiner, *Lonely at the Top: The High Cost of Men's Success*. New York: Palgrave Macmillan, 2011.

24   Thomas Hildebrandt, Justine Lai, James Langenbucher, Melanie Schneider, Rachel Yehuda, and Donald Pfaff, "The Diagnostic Dilemma of Pathological Appearance and Performance Enhancing Drug Use." *Drug and Alcohol Dependence* 114, no. 1 (2011): 1–11.

25   Thomas Hildebrandt, James Langenbucher, Sasha Carr, Pilar Sanjuan, and Steff Park, "Predicting Intentions for Long-Term Anabolic-Androgenic Steroid Use Among Men: A Covariance Structure Model." *Psychology of Addictive Behaviors* 20, no. 3 (2006): 234–40.

26   Thomas Hildebrandt et al., "The Diagnostic Dilemma of Pathological Appearance and Performance Enhancing Drug Use."

27   Brenda Goodman, "Wrestler Killed Wife and Son, Then Himself." *New York Times*, June 27, 2007.

28   Anahad O'Connor, "Wrestler Found to Have Taken Testosterone." *New York Times*, July 18, 2007.

29   Associated Press, "Benoit's Doctor Sentenced." *New York Times*, May 13, 2009.

30   D. Catherine Walker, Drew A. Anderson, and Thomas Hildebrandt, "Body Checking Behaviors in Men." *Body Image* 6, no. 3 (2009): 164–70.

31   Lauren Alfano, Thomas Hildebrandt, Katie Bannon, Catherine Walker, and Kate Walton, "The Impact of Gender on the Assessment of Body Checking Behavior." *Body Image* 8, no. 1 (2011): 20–5.

32   Thomas Hildebrandt, Jim Langenbucher, and David G. Schlundt, "Muscularity Concerns Among Men: Development of Attitudinal and Perceptual Measures." *Body Image* 1, no. 2 (2004): 169–81.

33   Richard Leit, James Gray, and Harrison Pope Jr., "The Media's Representation of the Ideal Male Body: A Cause for Muscle Dysmorphia?" *International Journal of Eating Disorders* 31, no. 3 (2002): 334–8.

34   Courtney Pope, Harrison Pope, William Menard, Christina

Fay, Roberto Olivardia, and Katherine Phillips, "Clinical Features of Muscle Dysmorphia Among Males with Body Dysmorphic Disorder." *Body Image* 2, no. 4 (2005): 395–400.

35 Donald McCreary, Thomas Hildebrandt, Leslie Heinberg, Michael Boroughs, and J. Kevin Thompson, "A Review of Body Image Influences on Men's Fitness Goals and Supplement Use." *American Journal of Men's Health* 1, no. 4 (2007): 307–16.

36 Courtney Pope et al., "Clinical Features of Muscle Dysmorphia Among Males with Body Dysmorphic Disorder."

37 Thomas Hildebrandt, David Schlundt, James Langenbucher, and Tammy Chung, "Presence of Muscle Dysmorphia Symptomology Among Male Weightlifters." *Comprehensive Psychiatry* 47, no. 2 (2006): 127–35.

38 Thomas Hildebrandt, Lauren Alfano, and James Langenbucher, "Body Image Disturbance in 1,000 Male Appearance and Performance Enhancing Drug Users." *Journal of Psychiatric Research* 44, no. 13 (2010): 841–6.

39 John Prescott tells of his battle with bulimia (2008). Retrieved August 1, 2012, from http://www.telegraph.co.uk/news/politics /labour/1896154/John-Prescott-tells-of-his-battle-with-bulimia .html.

CHAPTER 5: THE CHANGING CONTEXT OF EATING DISORDERS

1 Matt McGowan, "What's Not on the Menu?," University of Arkansas, http://researchfrontiers.uark.edu/6145.php.

2 Karen Hamrick, "How Much Time Do Americans Spend Eating?" In *USDA Blog*: United States Department of Agriculture, 2011.

3 Eric Schlosser, "Fast Food Nation: The Dark Side of the All-American Meal." *New York Times*, http://www.nytimes.com /books/first/s/schlosser-fast.html?_r=2.

4 Marni Jameson, "Eating at Restaurants Boosts Risk of Obesity, Experts Warn." *Orlando Sentinel*, July 4, 2011.

5 United States Department of Agriculture, "Choosemyplate .Gov," http://www.choosemyplate.gov.

6 North Iowa Municipal Electric Cooperative Association (NIMECA), "Take a Look at Your Diet," http://www.nimeca .com/aspx/News.aspx?NewsID=570.

7 CBS News, *The Early Show,* "How Americans Eat Today."
   January 12, 2010.

8 Brian Wansink and Collin Payne, "The Joy of Cooking Too
   Much: 70 Years of Calorie Increases in Classic Recipes."
   Annals of Internal Medicine 150, no. 4 (2009): 291–2.

9 Chelsey Keeler, "70 Years of Calorie Increases in Classic
   Recipes," http://foodpsychology.cornell.edu/outreach/joy-of
   -cooking.html.

10 Elizabeth Ward, "Sugar Shock: Should Your Sweet Tooth Be
   Regulated?" In "Nutrition Nation," *USAToday,* February 6,
   2012.

11 Sharon Johnson, Paulelda Gilbert, Ruth Litchfield, and Diane
   Nelson, "Soft Drink Portions Make a Difference." Iowa State
   University, Ames, Iowa, 2009.

12 Grace Ibay, "Foods High in Added Sugar." Livestrong.com,
   http://www.livestrong.com/article/350500-foods-high-in-added
   -sugar.

13 Ibid.

14 CBS News, *The Early Show,* "How Americans Eat Today."

15 BodyEcology, "The Six Thousand Hidden Dangers of Processed Foods (and What to Choose Instead)." In *BodyEcology,*
   2007.

16 Sanjay Gupta, "If We Are What We Eat, Americans Are Corn
   and Soy." *CNN Health,* 2007, and http://articles.cnn.com/2007
   -09-22/health/kd.gupta.column_1.

17 Michael Pollan, *The Omnivore's Dilemma: A Natural History of
   Four Meals.* New York: Penguin, 2007.

18 Food Insight, "2009 Food & Health Survey: Consumer Attitudes Toward Food, Nutrition and Health," ed. International
   Food Information Council Foundation, 2009.

19 Joseph Calamia, "Fast Food Nation: Americans Cook Less
   than Any Developed Country," http://www.lifeslittlemysteries.
   com/1362-average-american-life-study.html.

20 Lance Gay, "Family Dinners of Yore Are Gone for Sure," http://
   www.Seattlepi.Com/Lifestyle/Food/Article/Family-Dinners-of
   -Yore-Are-Gone-for-Sure-1195808.php. *seattlepi.com,* February
   14, 2006.

21 Timi Gustafson, "Despite of [sic] the Obesity Crisis, the
   Eating Habits of Most Americans Remain Unchanged." In
   seattlepi.com. Seattle, 2011.

22   Foodnetwork.com, *Sandra Lee Semi-Homemade Cooking,* 2012.

23   Tara Parker-Pope, "The Pedometer Test: Americans Take Fewer Steps." *New York Times,* October 19, 2010.

24   David Bassett Jr., Holly Wyatt, Helen Thompson, John Peters, and James Hill, "Pedometer-Measured Physical Activity and Health Behaviors in U.S. Adults." *Medicine and Science in Sports and Exercise* 42, no. 10 (2010): 1819–25.

25   Tara Parker-Pope, "Less Active at Work, Americans Have Packed on Pounds." *New York Times,* May 25, 2011.

26   Timothy Church, Diana Thomas, Catrine Tudor-Locke, Peter Katzmarzyk, Conrad Earnest, Ruben Rodarte, Corby Martin, Steven Blair, and Claude Bouchard, "Trends over 5 Decades in U.S. Occupation-Related Physical Activity and Their Associations with Obesity." *PloS One* 6, no. 5 (2011): e19657.

27   Charles E. Matthews, Kong Chen, Patty Freedson, Maciej Buchowski, Bettina Beech, Russell Pate, and Richard Troiano, "Amount of Time Spent in Sedentary Behaviors in the United States, 2003–2004." *American Journal of Epidemiology* 167, no. 7 (2008): 875–81.

28   Centers for Disease Control and Prevention, "How Much Physical Activity Do Adults Need?," ed. Centers for Disease Control and Prevention. Atlanta, 2011.

29   Genevieve Healy, David Dunstan, Jo Salmon, Ester Cerin, Jonathan Shaw, Paul Zimmet, and Neville Owen, "Breaks in Sedentary Time: Beneficial Associations with Metabolic Risk." *Diabetes Care* 31, no. 4 (2008): 661–6.

30   Barry Popkin, "The Nutrition Transition and Obesity in the Developing World." *Journal of Nutrition* 131, no. 3 (2001): 871S–73S; Barry Popkin, "An Overview on the Nutrition Transition and Its Health Implications: The Bellagio Meeting." *Public Health Nutrition* 5, no. 1A (2002): 93–103; and Barry Popkin and Penny Gordon-Larsen, "The Nutrition Transition: Worldwide Obesity Dynamics and Their Determinants." *International Journal of Obesity and Related Metabolic Disorders* 28 Suppl. 3 (2004): S2–9.

31   Manfred Fichter, M. Elton, L. Sourdi, Siegfried Weyerer, and G. Koptagel-Ilal, "Anorexia Nervosa in Greek and Turkish Adolescents." *European Archives of Psychiatry and Neurological Sciences* 237, no. 4 (1988): 200–8.

32   Anne Becker, Rebecca Burwell, Stephen Gilman, David
     Herzog, and Paul Hamburg, "Eating Behaviours and Attitudes
     Following Prolonged Exposure to Television Among Ethnic
     Fijian Adolescent Girls." *British Journal of Psychiatry* 180
     (2002): 509–14; and Anne Becker, Kristen Fay, Jessica Agnew-
     Blais, A. Nisha Khan, Ruth Striegel-Moore, and Stephen
     Gilman, "Social Network Media Exposure and Adolescent
     Eating Pathology in Fiji." *British Journal of Psychiatry* 198, no. 1
     (2011): 43–50.

33   Nobuo Kiriike, Toshihiko Nagata, Kumiko Sirata, and Naoki
     Yamamoto, "Are Young Women in Japan at High Risk for
     Eating Disorders? Decreased BMI in Young Females from 1960
     to 1995." *Psychiatry and Clinical Neurosciences* 52, no. 3 (1998):
     279–81.

34   Christine C. Iijima Hall, "Asian Eyes: Body Image and Eating
     Disorders of Asian and Asian American Women." *Eating Disor-
     ders: The Journal of Treatment & Prevention* 3, no. 1 (1995):
     8–19.

35   Akiko Fujita, "Diminishing Waistlines, a Japanese Health
     Problem." *ABC News*, February 17, 2012.

36   David B. Mumford, Andrew Whitehouse, and Margaret Platts,
     "Sociocultural Correlates of Eating Disorders Among Asian
     Schoolgirls in Bradford." *British Journal of Psychiatry* 158
     (1991): 222–8.

37   Sudhir Kumar Khandelwal, Pratap Sharan, and S. Saxena,
     "Eating Disorders: An Indian Perspective." *International
     Journal of Social Psychiatry* 41, no. 2 (1995): 132–46.

38   Jaehee Jung and Gordon Forbes, "Body Dissatisfaction and
     Disordered Eating Among College Women in China, South
     Korea, and the United States: Contrasting Predictions from
     Sociocultural and Feminist Theories." *Psychology of Women
     Quarterly* 31 (2007): 381–93.

39   Hans Hoek, Peter van Harten, Daphne van Hoeken, and Ezra
     Susser, "Lack of Relation Between Culture and Anorexia
     Nervosa: Results of an Incidence Study on Curaçao." *New
     England Journal of Medicine* 338, no. 17 (1998): 1231–2; and
     Melanie Katzman, Karin Hermans, Daphne Van Hoeken, and
     Hans Hoek, "Not Your 'Typical Island Woman': Anorexia
     Nervosa Is Reported Only in Subcultures in Curaçao."
     Culture, Medicine and Psychiatry 28, no. 4 (2004): 463–92.

40 The Jackson Laboratory, "Jax Mice Strains," http://jaxmice.jax
.org/list/cat481365.html.

41 Wendy Foulds Mathes, David Aylor, Darla Miller, Gary
Churchill, Elissa Chesler, Fernando Pardo de Villena, David
Threadgill, and Daniel Pomp, "Architecture of Energy Balance
Traits in Emerging Lines of the Collaborative Cross." *American Journal of Physiology, Endocrinology and Metabolism* 300,
no. 6 (2011): E1124–34.

42 Gina Kolata, "Brown Fat, Triggered by Cold or Exercise, May
Yield a Key to Weight Control." *New York Times*, January 24, 2012.

43 Véronique Ouellet, Sébastien M. Labbe, Denis P. Blondin,
Serge Phoenix, Brigitte Guerin, François Haman, Eric
Turcotte, Denis Richard, and André Carpentier. "Brown
Adipose Tissue Oxidative Metabolism Contributes to Energy
Expenditure During Acute Cold Exposure in Humans."
Journal of Clinical Investigation 122, no. 2 (2012): 545–52.

44 Ponotus Boström, Jun Wu, Mark Jedrychowski, Anisna Korde,
Li Ye, James Lo, Kyle Rasbach, Elisabeth Boström, Jang
Choi, Jonathan Z. Long, Shingo Kajimura, Maria Zingaretti,
Birgitte Vind, Hua Tu, Saverio Cinti, Kurt Højlund, Steven Gygi,
and Bruce Spiegelman, "A Pgc1-Alpha-Dependent Myokine
That Drives Brown-Fat-Like Development of White Fat and
Thermogenesis." *Nature* 481, no. 7382 (2012): 463–8.

45 Katherine Flegal, Margaret Carroll, Carroll Ogden, and
Clifford Johnson, "Prevalence and Trends in Obesity among
US Adults, 1999–2000." *Journal of the American Medical
Association* 288, no. 14 (2002): 1723–7.

46 National Sleep Foundation, "2002 'Sleep in America' Poll."
Washington, DC: 2002; and Daniel Kripke, Ruth Simons,
Lawrence Garfinkel, and F. Cuyler Hammond, "Short and
Long Sleep and Sleeping Pills. Is Increased Mortality Associated?" *Archives of General Psychiatry* 36, no. 1 (1979): 103–16.

47 James Gangwisch, Dolores Malaspina, Bernadette Boden-
Albala, and Steven Heymsfield, "Inadequate Sleep as a Risk
Factor for Obesity: Analyses of the NHANES I." *Sleep* 28, no.
10 (2005): 1289–96.

48 Kristen Knutson, Karine Spiegel, Plamen Penev, and Eve Van
Cauter. "The Metabolic Consequences of Sleep Deprivation."
Sleep Medicine Reviews 11, no. 3 (2007): 163–78; Jean-Philippe
Chaput, Jean-Pierre Despres, Claude Bouchard, and Angelo

Tremblay. "Short Sleep Duration Is Associated with Reduced Leptin Levels and Increased Adiposity: Results from the Quebec Family Study." *Obesity* 15, no. 1 (2007): 253–61; and Karine Spiegel, Esra Tasali, Plamen Penev, and Eve Van Cauter, "Brief Communication: Sleep Curtailment in Healthy Young Men Is Associated with Decreased Leptin Levels, Elevated Ghrelin Levels, and Increased Hunger and Appetite." *Annals of Internal Medicine* 141, no. 11 (2004): 846–50.

49 Sara Trace, Laura Thornton, Cristin Runfola, Paul Lichtenstein, Nancy Pedersen, and Cynthia Bulik, "Sleep Problems Are Associated with Binge Eating in Women." *International Journal of Eating Disorders* 45, no. 5 (2012): 695–703.

50 Annie Artiga, Jason Viana, Carlos Maldonado, Pamela Chandler-Laney, Kimberly Oswald, and Mary Boggiano, "Body Composition and Endocrine Status of Long-Term Stress-Induced Binge-Eating Rats." *Physiology & Behavior* 91, no. 4 (2007): 424–31; Elissa Epel, Rachel Lapidus, Bruce McEwen, and Kelly Brownell, "Stress May Add Bite to Appetite in Women: A Laboratory Study of Stress-Induced Cortisol and Eating Behavior." *Psychoneuroendocrinology* 26, no. 1 (2001): 37–49; Alexandros N. Vgontzas, Hung-Mo Lin, Maria Papaliaga, Susan Calhoun, Antonio Vela-Bueno, George P. Chrousos, and Edward O. Bixler, "Short Sleep Duration and Obesity: The Role of Emotional Stress and Sleep Disturbances." *International Journal of Obesity* 32, no. 5 (2008): 801–9.

51 Emily Newman, Daryl O'Connor, and Mark Conner, "Daily Hassles and Eating Behaviour: The Role of Cortisol Reactivity Status." *Psychoneuroendocrinology* 32, no. 2 (2007): 125–32.

52 Walmir Coutinho, Rodrigo Moreira, Camila Spagnol, and Jose Appolinario, "Does Binge Eating Disorder Alter Cortisol Secretion in Obese Women?" *Eating Behaviors* 8, no. 1 (2007): 59–64.

53 Marcella Balbo, Rachel Leproult, and Eve Van Cauter, "Impact of Sleep and Its Disturbances on Hypothalamo-Pituitary-Adrenal Axis Activity." *International Journal of Endocrinology* (2010): 759234.

54 Tammy Root, Laura Thornton, Anna Karin Lindroos, Albert J. Stunkard, Paul Lichtenstein, Nancy L. Pedersen, Finn Rasmussen, and Cynthia Bulik, "Shared and Unique Genetic and Environmental Influences on Binge Eating and Night

Eating: A Swedish Twin Study." *Eating Behaviors* 11, no. 2 (2010): 92–8.

CHAPTER 6: GENES AND ENVIRONMENT AT ANY AGE

1 Andrew Jeremy Wakefield, Simon Murch, Andrew Anthony, John Linnell, David M. Casson, Moshin Malik, Mark Berelowitz, Amar Dhillon, Mike Ahomson, Peter Harvey, Alan Valentine, Susan Davies, and John Walker-Smith, "Ileal-Lymphoid-Nodular Hyperplasia, Non-Specific Colitis, and Pervasive Developmental Disorder in Children." *Lancet* 351, no. 9103 (1998): 637–41.

2 Fiona Godlee, Jane Smith, and Harvey Marcovitch, "Wakefield's Article Linking MMR Vaccine and Autism Was Fraudulent." *British Medical Journal* 342 (2011): c7452.

3 Chris Mooney, "Why Does the Vaccine/Autism Controversy Live On?" *Discover Magazine*, June 2009.

4 Jenny McCarthy, "Generation Rescue: Hope for Recovery," http://www.generationrescue.org.

5 Gloria Steinem, "Women's Liberation Aims to Free Men, Too." *Washington Post*, June 7, 1970.

6 Salvador Minuchin, Bernice Rosman, and Lester Baker, *Psychosomatic Families: Anorexia Nervosa in Context.* Cambridge, MA: Harvard University Press, 1978.

7 Bruno Bettelheim, *The Empty Fortress: Infantile Autism and the Birth of the Self.* New York: The Free Press, 1967.

8 Frieda Fromm-Reichmann, "Notes on the Development of Treatment of Schizophrenics by Psychoanalysis and Psychotherapy." *Psychiatry* 11, no. 3 (1948): 263–73.

9 Gregory Bateson, Don Jackson, Jay Haley, and John Weakland, "Toward a Theory of Schizophrenia." *Behavioral Science* 1, no. 4 (1956): 251–64.

10 Marsha Marcus, Joyce Bromberger, Hsio-Lan Wei, Charlotte Brown, and Howard M. Kravitz, "Prevalence and Selected Correlates of Eating Disorder Symptoms Among a Multiethnic Community Sample of Midlife Women." *Annals of Behavioral Medicine* 33, no. 3 (2007): 269–77; Ruth Striegel-Moore, Faith Dohm, Helena Kraemer, George Schreiber, C. Barr Taylor, and Stephen R. Daniels, "Risk Factors for Binge-Eating

Disorders: An Exploratory Study." *International Journal of Eating Disorders* 40, no. 6 (2007): 481–7; and Ruth Striegel-Moore, Faith-Anne Dohm, Helena Kraemer, C. Barr Taylor, Stephen Daniels, Patricia Crawford, and George Schreiber, "Eating Disorders in White and Black Women." *American Journal of Psychiatry* 160, no. 7 (2003): 1326–31.

11   Anne Becker, Debra Franko, Alexandra Speck, and David Herzog, "Ethnicity and Differential Access to Care for Eating Disorder Symptoms." *International Journal of Eating Disorders* 33, no. 2 (2003): 205–12.

12   Lisa Lilenfeld, Walter Kaye, Catherine Greeno, Kathleen Merikangas, Katherine Plotnikov, Christine Pollice, Radhika Rao, Michael Strober, Cynthia Bulik, and Linda Nagy, "A Controlled Family Study of Restricting Anorexia and Bulimia Nervosa: Comorbidity in Probands and Disorders in First-Degree Relatives." *Archives of General Psychiatry* 55, no.7 (1998): 603–10; and Michael Strober, Roberta Freeman, Carlyn Lampert, Jane Diamond, and Walter Kaye, "Controlled Family Study of Anorexia Nervosa and Bulimia Nervosa: Evidence of Shared Liability and Transmission of Partial Syndromes." *American Journal of Psychiatry* 157, no. 3 (2000): 393–401.

13   James Hudson, Justine Lalonde, Lindsay Pindyck, Cynthia Bulik, Scott Crow, Susan McElroy, Nan Laird, Ming Tsuang, Norman Rosenthal, and Harrison Pope, "Familial Aggregation of Binge-Eating Disorder." *Archives of General Psychiatry* 63, no. 3 (2006): 313–9.

14   Cynthia Bulik, Laura Thornton, Tammy Root, Emily Pisetsky, Paul Lichtenstein, and Nancy L. Pedersen, "Understanding the Relation between Anorexia Nervosa and Bulimia Nervosa in a Swedish National Twin Sample." *Biological Psychiatry* 67, no. 1 (2010): 71–7; Kelly Klump, Kathryn Miller, Pamela Keel, Matthew McGue, and William Iacono, "Genetic and Environmental Influences on Anorexia Nervosa Syndromes in a Population-Based Twin Sample." *Psychological Medicine* 31, no. 4 (2001): 737–40; Cynthia Bulik, Patrick Sullivan, Tracey Wade, and Kenneth Kendler, "Twin Studies of Eating Disorders: A Review." *International Journal of Eating Disorders* 27, no. 1 (2000): 1–20.

15   Kristin Javaras, Nan Laird, Ted Reichborn-Kjennerud, Cynthia Bulik, Harrison Pope Jr., and James Hudson, "Familiality and Heritability of Binge Eating Disorder: Results of a

Case-Control Family Study and a Twin Study." *International Journal of Eating Disorders* 41, no. 2 (2008): 174–9; Ted Reichborn-Kjennerud, Cynthia Bulik, Kristian Tambs, and Jennifer Harris, "Genetic and Environmental Influences on Binge Eating in the Absence of Compensatory Behaviours: A Population-Based Twin Study." *International Journal of Eating Disorders* 36, no. 3 (2004): 307–14.

16 National Institute of General Medical Sciences, "The Genetic Architecture of Complex Traits Workshop." National Institutes of Health, 1998.

17 Thomas Scioscia, Cynthia Bulik, James Levenson, and Donald Kirby, "Anorexia Nervosa in a 38-Year-Old Woman 2 Years after Gastric Bypass Surgery." *Psychosomatics* 40, no. 1 (1999): 86–8.

18 Joanna Marino, Troy Ertelt, Kathy Lancaster, Kristine Steffen, Lisa Peterson, Martina de Zwaan, and James Mitchell, "The Emergence of Eating Pathology After Bariatric Surgery: A Rare Outcome with Important Clinical Implications." *International Journal of Eating Disorders* 45, no. 2 (2012): 179–84.

19 Sharon Alger-Mayer, Carl Rosati, John Polimeni, and Margaret Malone, "Preoperative Binge Eating Status and Gastric Bypass Surgery: A Long-Term Outcome Study." *Obesity Surgery* 19, no. 2 (2009): 139–45; Jarol Boan, Ronette Kolotkin, Eric Westman, Ross McMahon, and John Grant, "Binge Eating, Quality of Life and Physical Activity Improve After Roux-En-Y Gastric Bypass for Morbid Obesity." *Obesity Surgery* 14, no. 3 (2004): 341–8; Margaret Malone and Sharon Alger-Mayer, "Binge Status and Quality of Life After Gastric Bypass Surgery: A One-Year Study." *Obesity Research* 12, no. 3 (2004): 473–81.

CHAPTER 7: PARTNERS SUFFER

1 Mildred Maxwell, Laura Thornton, Tammy Root, Andrea Pinheiro, Michael Strober, Harry Brandt, Steven Crawford, Scott Crow, Manfred Fichter, Katherine Halmi, Craig Johnson, Allan Kaplan, Pamela Keel, Kelly Klump, Maria LaVia, James Mitchell, Katherine Plotnicov, Alessandro Rotondo, D. Blake Woodside, Wade Berrettini, Walter Kaye, and Cynthia Bulik, "Life Beyond the Eating Disorder: Education, Relationships, and Reproduction." *International Journal of Eating Disorders* 44, no. 3 (2011): 225–32.

2   Ruth Striegel, Richard Bedrosian, Chun Wang, and Steven
     Schwartz, "Why Men Should Be Included in Research on
     Binge Eating: Results from a Comparison of Psychosocial
     Impairment in Men and Women." *International Journal of
     Eating Disorders* 45, no. 2 (2012): 233–40.
3   Matthew Feldman and Ilan Meyer, "Eating Disorders in
     Diverse Lesbian, Gay, and Bisexual Populations." *International
     Journal of Eating Disorders* 40, no. 3 (2007): 218–26.
4   Debora Bussolotti, Fernando Fernández-Aranda, Raquel
     Solano, Susanna Jiménez-Murcia, Vicente Turon, and Julio
     Vallejo, "Marital Status and Eating Disorders: An Analysis of
     Its Relevance." *Journal of Psychosomatic Research* 53, no. 6
     (2002): 1139–45.
5   Dorothy Van Buren and Donald Williamson, "Marital Rela-
     tionships and Conflict Resolution Skills of Bulimics." *Interna-
     tional Journal of Eating Disorders* 7, no. 6 (1988): 735–41; D.
     Blake Woodside, Jan Lackstrom, and Lorie Shekter-Wolfson,
     "Marriage in Eating Disorders: Comparisons Between Patients
     and Spouses and Changes over the Course of Treatment."
     Journal of Psychosomatic Research 49, no. 3 (2000): 165–8.
6   Michael Friedman, Amy Dixon, Kelly Brownell, Mark Whis-
     man, and Denise Wilfley, "Marital Status, Marital Satisfac-
     tion, and Body Image Dissatisfaction." *International Journal of
     Eating Disorders* 26, no. 1 (1999): 81–5.
7   Mark Whisman, Anastasia Dementyeva, Donald Baucom, and
     Cynthia Bulik, "Marital Functioning and Binge Eating
     Disorder in Married Women." *International Journal of Eating
     Disorders* 45, no. 3 (2012): 385–9.
8   Benjamin Karney and Thomas Bradbury, "The Longitudinal
     Course of Marital Quality and Stability: A Review of Theory,
     Methods, and Research." *Psychological Bulletin* 118, no. 1
     (1995): 3–34.
9   Stephen Van den Broucke and Walter Vandereycken, "An-
     orexia and Bulimia Nervosa in Married Patients: A Review."
     Comprehensive Psychiatry 29, no. 2 (1988): 165–73.
10   Ralphe Grabhorn, Hanna Stenner, Johannes Kaufbold, Gerd
     Overbeck, and Ullrich Stangier, "[Shame and Social Anxiety
     in Anorexia and Bulimia Nervosa]." *Zeitschrift für Psychosoma-
     tische Medizin und Psychotherapie* 51, no. 2 (2005): 179–93;
     Madhulika Gupta, Aditya Gupta, Nicholas Schork, and Gena
     Watteel, "Perceived Touch Deprivation and Body Image: Some

Observations Among Eating Disordered and Non-Clinical Subjects." *Journal of Psychosomatic Research* 39, no. 4 (1995): 459–64.

11 Jin Raboch and František Faltus, "Sexuality of Women with Anorexia Nervosa." *Acta Psychiatrica Scandinavica* 84, no. 1 (1991): 9–11.

12 Andrea Pinheiro, Thomas Raney, Laura Thornton, Manfred Fichter, Wade Berrettini, David Goldman, Katherine Halmi, Allan Kaplan, Michael Strober, Janet Treasure, D. Blake Woodside, Walter Kaye, and Cynthia Bulik, "Sexual Functioning in Women with Eating Disorders." *International Journal of Eating Disorders* 43, no. 2 (2010): 123–129.

13 C. Don Morgan, Michael Wiederman, and Tamara Pryor, "Sexual Functioning and Attitudes of Eating-Disordered Women: A Follow-up Study." *Journal of Sex and Marital Therapy* 21, no. 2 (1995): 67–77.

14 Andrea Poyastro Pinheiro, Laura Thornton, Katherine Plotonicov, Federica Tozzi, Kelly Klump, Wade Berrettini, Harry Brandt, Steven Crawford, Scott Crow, Manfred Fichter, David Goldman, Katherine Halmi, Craig Johnson, Allan Kaplan, Pamela Keel, Maria LaVia, James Mitchell, Alessandro Rotondo, Michael Strober, Janet Treasure, D. Blake Woodside, Ann Von Holle, Robert Hamer, Walter Kaye, and Cynthia Bulik, "Patterns of Menstrual Disturbance in Eating Disorders." *International Journal of Eating Disorders* 40, no. 5 (2007): 424–34.

15 Michael Wiederman, Tamara Pryor, and C. Don Morgan, "The Sexual Experience of Women Diagnosed with Anorexia Nervosa or Bulimia Nervosa." *International Journal of Eating Disorders* 19, no. 2 (1996): 109–18.

16 Peter Beumont, Suzanne Abraham, and Kathleen Simson, "The Psychosexual Histories of Adolescent Girls and Young Women with Anorexia Nervosa." *Psychological Medicine* 11, no. 1 (1981): 131–40.

17 John Morgan, John Hubert Lacey, and Fiona Reid, "Anorexia Nervosa: Changes in Sexuality During Weight Restoration." *Psychosomatic Medicine* 61, no. 4 (1999): 541–5.

18 Paolo Santonastaso, Diego Saccon, and Angela Favaro, "Burden and Psychiatric Symptoms on Key Relatives of Patients with Eating Disorders: A Preliminary Study." *Eating and Weight Disorders* 2, no. 1 (1997): 44–8.

19   Janet Treasure, Tara Murphy, George Szmukler, Gill Todd, Kay Gavan, and J. Joyce, "The Experience of Caregiving for Severe Mental Illness: A Comparison Between Anorexia Nervosa and Psychosis." *Social Psychiatry and Psychiatric Epidemiology* 36, no. 7 (2001): 343–7.

20   Jenna Whitney, Joanna Murray, Kay Gavan, Gill Todd, Wendy Whitaker, and Janet Treasure, "Experience of Caring for Someone with Anorexia Nervosa: Qualitative Study." *British Journal of Psychiatry* 187 (2005): 444–9.

21   Roel Hermans, Anna Lichtwarck-Aschoff, Kirsten Bevelander, C. Peter Herman, Junilla Larsen, and Rutger Engels, "Mimicry of Food Intake: The Dynamic Interplay Between Eating Companions." *PloS One* 7, no. 2 (2012): e31027.

CHAPTER 8: PREGNANCY, CHILDBIRTH, AND EATING DISORDERS

1   Andrea Poyastro Pinheiro, Laura Thornton, Katherine Plotonicov, Federica Tozzi, Kelly Klump, Wade Berrettini, Harry Brandt, Steven Crawford, Scott Crow, Manfred Fichter, David Goldman, Katherine Halmi, Craig Johnson, Allan Kaplan, Pamela Keel, Maria LaVia, James Mitchell, Alessandro Rotondo, Michael Strober, Janet Treasure, D. Blake Woodside, Ann Von Holle, Robert M. Hamer, Walter Kaye, and Cynthia Bulik, "Patterns of Menstrual Disturbance in Eating Disorders." *International Journal of Eating Disorders* 40, no. 5 (2007): 424–34; and Kelly Gendall, Peter Joyce, Frances Carter, Virginia McIntosh, Jennifer Jordan, and Cynthia Bulik, "The Psychobiology and Diagnostic Significance of Amenorrhea in Patients with Anorexia Nervosa." *Fertility and Sterility* 85, no. 5 (2006): 1531–5.

2   Melissa Freizinger, Debra Franko, Marie Dacey, Barbara Okun, and Alice Domar, "The Prevalence of Eating Disorders in Infertile Women." *Fertility and Sterility* 93, no. 1 (2010): 72–8; and Donna Stewart, G. Erlick Robinson, David Goldbloom, and Charlene Wright, "Infertility and Eating Disorders." *American Journal of Obstetrics and Gynecology* 163, no. 4 (1990): 1196–99.

3   Abigail Easter, Janet Treasure, and Nadia Micali, "Fertility and Prenatal Attitudes Towards Pregnancy in Women with Eating Disorders: Results from the Avon Longitudinal Study

of Parents and Children." *British Journal of Obstetrics and Gynaecology* 118, no. 12 (2011): 1491–8.

4 Scott Crow, Paul Thuras, Pamela Keel, and James Mitchell, "Long-Term Menstrual and Reproductive Function in Patients with Bulimia Nervosa." *American Journal of Psychiatry* 159, no. 6 (2002): 1048–50.

5 Chiara Sbaragli, Giuseppe Morgante, Arianna Goracci, Tara Hofkens, Vincenzo De Leo, and Paolo Castrogiovanni, "Infertility and Psychiatric Morbidity." *Fertility and Sterility* 90, no. 6 (2008): 2107–11.

6 Markus Jokela, Mika Kivimaki, Marko Elovainio, Jormas Viikari, Olli T. Raitakari, and Liisa Keltikangas-Jarvinen, "Body Mass Index in Adolescence and Number of Children in Adulthood." *Epidemiology* 18, no. 5 (2007): 599–606.

7 Stergios Moschos, Jean Chan, and Christos Mantzoros, "Leptin and Reproduction: A Review." *Fertility and Sterility* 77, no. 3 (2002): 433–44.

8 Cynthia Bulik, Elizabeth Hoffman, Ann Von Holle, Leila Torgersen, Camilla Stoltenberg, and Ted Reichborn-Kjennerud, "Unplanned Pregnancy in Women with Anorexia Nervosa." *Obstetrics and Gynecology* 116, no. 5 (2010): 1136–40.

9 Abigail Easter et al., "Fertility and Prenatal Attitudes Towards Pregnancy in Women with Eating Disorders."

10 John Morgan, J. Hubert Lacey, and Elaine Chung, "Risk of Postnatal Depression, Miscarriage, and Preterm Birth in Bulimia Nervosa: Retrospective Controlled Study." *Psychosomatic Medicine* 68, no. 3 (2006): 487–92.

11 Christopher Fairburn, Alan Stein, and Rosemary Jones, "Eating Habits and Eating Disorders During Pregnancy." *Psychosomatic Medicine* 54, no. 6 (1992): 665–72; Scott Crow, W. Stewart Agras, Ross Crosby, Katherine Halmi, and James Mitchell, "Eating Disorder Symptoms in Pregnancy: A Prospective Study." *International Journal of Eating Disorders* 41, no. 3 (2008): 277–9; and Nadia Micali, Janet Treasure, and Emily Simonoff, "Eating Disorders Symptoms in Pregnancy: A Longitudinal Study of Women with Recent and Past Eating Disorders and Obesity." *Journal of Psychosomatic Research* 63, no. 3 (2007): 297–303.

12 Linda Lewis and Daniel Le Grange, "The Experience and Impact of Pregnancy in Bulimia Nervosa: A Series of Case Studies." *European Eating Disorders Review* 2 (1994): 93–105.

13   Sheila Namir, Kenneth Melman, and Joel Yager, "Pregnancy in
     Restrictor-Type Anorexia Nervosa: A Study of Six Women."
     International Journal of Eating Disorders 5, no. 5 (1986):
     837–45.
14   Food and Nutrition Board Institute of Medicine, "Dietary
     Reference Intakes for Energy, Carbohydrates, Fiber, Fat, Fatty
     Acids, Cholesterol, Protein and Amino Acids." Washington,
     DC: National Academy Press, 2002.
15   Food and Nutrition Board Institute of Medicine. "Dietary
     Reference Intakes for Thiamin, Riboflavin, Niacin, Vitamin
     B_6, Folate, Vitamin B_{12}, Pantothenic Acid, Biotin, and Cho-
     line." Washington, DC: National Academy Press, 1998.
16   Anna Maria Siega-Riz, Margarete Haugen, Helle Meltzer, Ann
     Von Holle, Robert M. Hamer, Leila Torgersen, Cecilie Knoph
     Berg, Ted Reichborn-Kjennerud, and Cynthia Bulik, "Nutrient
     and Food Group Intakes of Women with and without Bulimia
     Nervosa and Binge Eating Disorder During Pregnancy."
     American Journal of Clinical Nutrition 87, no. 5 (2008):
     1346–55; and Nadia Micali and Janet Treasure, "Biological
     Effects of a Maternal Eating Disorder on Pregnancy and
     Foetal Development: A Review." *European Eating Disorders
     Review* 17, no. 6 (2009): 448–54.
17   Anna Olafsdottir, Gudrun Skuladottir, Inga Thorsdottir, Arnar
     Hauksson, and Laufey Steingrimsdottir, "Maternal Diet in
     Early and Late Pregnancy in Relation to Weight Gain."
     International Journal of Obesity 30, no. 3 (2006): 492–9.
18   Anna Maria Siega-Riz, Ann Von Holle, Margarete Haugen,
     Helle Meltzer, Robert Hamer, Leila Torgersen, Cecilie Knoph
     Berg, Ted Reichborn-Kjennerud, and Cynthia Bulik, "Gesta-
     tional Weight Gain of Women with Eating Disorders in the
     Norwegian Pregnancy Cohort." *International Journal of Eating
     Disorders* 44, no. 5 (2011): 428–34.
19   Cynthia Bulik, Ann Von Holle, Anna Maria Siega-Riz, Leila
     Torgersen, Kari Kviem Lie, Robert M. Hamer, Cecilie Knoph
     Berg, Patrick Sullivan, and Ted Reichborn-Kjennerud, "Birth
     Outcomes in Women with Eating Disorders in the Norwegian
     Mother and Child Cohort Study (Moba)." *International
     Journal of Eating Disorders* 42, no. 1 (2009): 9–18.
20   Lindsay H. Allen. "Multiple Micronutrients in Pregnancy and
     Lactation: An Overview." *American Journal of Clinical
     Nutrition* 81, no. 5 (2005): 1206S–12S.

21   Anna Maria Siega-Riz et al, "Nutrient and Food Group Intakes of Women with and without Bulimia Nervosa and Binge Eating Disorder During Pregnancy."

22   Jocilyn Dellava, Ann Von Holle, Leila Torgersen, Ted Reichborn-Kjennerud, Margarete Haugen, Helle Meltzer, and Cynthia Bulik, "Dietary Supplement Use Immediately Before and During Pregnancy in Norwegian Women with Eating Disorders." *International Journal of Eating Disorders* 44, no. 4 (2011): 325–32.

23   Raymond Lemberg and Jeanne Phillips, "The Impact of Pregnancy on Anorexia Nervosa and Bulimia." *International Journal of Eating Disorders* 8 (1989): 285–95; and Scott Crow, Pamela Keel, Paul Thuras, and James Mitchell, "Bulimia Symptoms and Other Risk Behaviors During Pregnancy in Women with Bulimia Nervosa." *International Journal of Eating Disorders* 36, no. 2 (2004): 220–3.

24   Ibid.

25   Katherine Davies and Jane Wardle, "Body Image and Dieting in Pregnancy." *Journal of Psychosomatic Research* 38, no. 8 (1994): 787–99.

26   Saloua Koubaa, Tore Hallstrom, Caroline Lindholm, and Angelica Hirschberg, "Pregnancy and Neonatal Outcomes in Women with Eating Disorders." *Obstetrics and Gynecology* 105, no. 2 (2005): 255–60.

27   Nadia Micali et al., "Eating Disorders Symptoms in Pregnancy."

28   Cynthia Bulik, Ann Von Holle, Robert Hamer, Cecilie Knoph Berg, Leila Torgersen, Per Magnus, Camilla Stoltenberg, Anna Maria Siega-Riz, Patrick Sullivan, and Ted Reichborn-Kjennerud. "Patterns of Remission, Continuation and Incidence of Broadly Defined Eating Disorders During Early Pregnancy in the Norwegian Mother and Child Cohort Study (Moba)." *Psychological Medicine* 37, no. 8 (2007): 1109–18.

29   Nadia Micali et al., "Eating Disorders Symptoms in Pregnancy."

30   Linda Lewis and Daniel Le Grange, "The Experience and Impact of Pregnancy in Bulimia Nervosa."

31   Leila Torgersen, Ann Von Holle, Cecilie Knoph Berg, Robert Hamer, Anna Maria Siega-Riz, Patrick Sullivan, Ted Reichborn-Kjennerud, and Cynthia Bulik, "Nausea and Vomiting of Pregnancy in Women with Bulimia Nervosa and EDNOS." *International Journal of Eating Disorders* 41, no.8 (2008): 722–27.

32   Elizabeth Hoffman, Stephanie Zerwas, and Cynthia Bulik, "Reproductive Issues in Anorexia Nervosa." *Expert Review of Obstetrics & Gynecology* 6, no. 4 (2011): 403–14.

33   Ibid.

34   Cynthia Bulik et al., "Patterns of Remission, Continuation and Incidence of Broadly Defined Eating Disorders During Early Pregnancy in the Norwegian Mother and Child Cohort Study (Moba)."

35   Ibid.

36   Alan Stein and Christopher Fairburn, "Eating Habits and Attitudes in the Postpartum Period." *Psychosomatic Medicine* 58, no. 4 (1996): 321–25.

37   Lorraine Walker and Jeanne Freeland-Graves, "Lifestyle Factors Related to Postpartum Weight Gain and Body Image in Bottle- and Breastfeeding Women." *Journal of Obstetric, Gynecologic, and Neonatal Nursing* 27, no. 2 (1998): 151–60.

38   Dwenda Gjerdingen, Patricia Fontaine, Scott Crow, Patricia McGovern, Bruce Center, and Michael Miner, "Predictors of Mothers' Postpartum Body Dissatisfaction." *Women & Health* 49, no. 6 (2009): 491–504.

39   Stephanie Zerwas, Ann Von Holle, Leila Torgersen, Eliana Perrin, Asheley Skinner, Lauren Reba-Harrelson, Camilla Stoltenberg, Ted Reichborn-Kjennerud, and Cynthia Bulik, "Patterns of Pregnancy and Post-Partum Weight Change in Mothers with Eating Disorders from the Norwegian Mother and Child Cohort Study (Moba)" (submitted).

40   Womenshealth.gov, "Depression During and After Pregnancy Fact Sheet." Office on Women's Health, http://www.womens health.gov/publications/our-publications/fact-sheet/depression -pregnancy.cfm.

41   Suzanne Mazzeo, Margarita Slof-Op't Landt, Ian Jones, Karen Mitchell, Kenneth Kendler, Michael Neale, Steven Aggen, and Cynthia Bulik, "Associations Among Postpartum Depression, Eating Disorders, and Perfectionism in a Population-Based Sample of Adult Women." *International Journal of Eating Disorders* 39, no. 3 (2006): 202–11.

42   Linda Smolak and Sarah Murnen, "A Meta-Analytic Examination of the Relationship Between Child Sexual Abuse and Eating Disorders." *International Journal of Eating Disorders* 31, no. 2 (2002): 136–50.

43   Samantha Meltzer-Brody, Stephanie Zerwas, Jane Leserman,

Ann Von Holle, Taylor Regis, and Cynthia Bulik, "Eating Disorders and Trauma History in Women with Perinatal Depression." *Journal of Women's Health* 20, no. 6 (2011): 863–70.

44   Leila Torgersen, E. Ystrom, Margarete Haugen, Helle Meltzer, Ann Von Holle, Cecilie Knoph Berg, Ted Reichborn-Kjennerud, and Cynthia Bulik, "Breastfeeding Practice in Mothers with Eating Disorders." *Maternal & Child Nutrition* 6, no. 3 (2010): 243–52.

45   Philip Mehler, Barbara Cleary, and Jennifer Gaudiani, "Osteoporosis in Anorexia Nervosa." *Eating Disorders* 19, no. 2 (2011): 194–202.

46   Donna Stewart, G. Erlick Robinson, David Goldbloom, and Charlene Wright, "Infertility and Eating Disorders." *American Journal of Obstetrics and Gynecology* 163, no. 4, pt. 1 (1990): 1196–9.

47   Meaghan Leddy, Candice Jones, Maria Morgan, and Jay Schulkin, "Eating Disorders and Obstetric-Gynecologic Care." *Journal of Women's Health* 18, no. 9 (2009): 1395–401.

48   Raymond Lemberg and Jeanne Phillips, "The Impact of Pregnancy on Anorexia Nervosa and Bulimia."

49   Kimberly Yonkers, Katherine Wisner, Donna Stewart, Tim Oberlander, Diana Dell, Nada Stotland, Susan Ramin, Linda Chaudron, and Charles Lockwood, "The Management of Depression During Pregnancy: A Report from the American Psychiatric Association and the American College of Obstetricians and Gynecologists." *Obstetrics and Gynecology* 114, no. 3 (2009): 703–13.

CHAPTER 9: PARENTING WITH AN EATING DISORDER

1   Ellyn Satter, "How to Feed Children," http://www.ellynsatter .com/how-to-feed-i-24.html.

2   Elizabeth Hoffman, Margaret Bentley, Robert M. Hamer, Eric Hodges, Dianne Ward, and Cynthia Bulik, "A Comparison of Infant and Toddler Feeding Practices of Mothers with and without Histories of Eating Disorders." *Maternal and Child Nutrition* (2012).

3   Robert Kenner, *Food, Inc.* 2008.

4   Victoria Spring and Cynthia Bulik, "Implicit Affect Toward

Food and Weight: A Neurocognitive Marker for Anorexia Nervosa?" (submitted).

5   Dewi Guardia, Léa Conversy, Renaud Jardri, Gilles Lafargue, Pierre Thomas, Vincent Dodin, Olivier Cottencin, Marion Luyat, "Imagining One's Own and Somebody Else's Actions: Dissociation in Anorexia Nervosa." *PLOSOne* 7, no. 8 (2012): e43241.

6   Addys Moreno and Mark Thelen, "Parental Factors Related to Bulimia Nervosa." *Addictive Behaviors* 18, no. 6 (1993): 681–9.

7   Deirde M. Kanakis and Mark Thelen, "Parental Variables Associated with Bulimia Nervosa." *Addictive Behaviors* 20, no. 4 (1995): 491–500.

8   Daniel DeNoon, "Parents, Kids, Doctors Balk at Talk About Weight." WebMD, http://www.webmd.com/parenting/news /20110914/parents-kids-doctors-balk-at-talk-about-weight.

9   Sheri Volger, Marion Vetter, Megan Dougherty, Eva Panigrahi, Rebecca Egner, Victoria Webb, J. Graham Thomas, David Sarwer, and Thomas Wadden, "Patients' Preferred Terms for Describing Their Excess Weight: Discussing Obesity in Clinical Practice." *Obesity* 20, no. 1 (2012): 147–50.

CHAPTER 10: MOTIVATORS FOR RECOVERY

1   Josie Geller, "How and When? The Ingredients of Change." In *Restoring Our Bodies, Reclaiming Our Lives: Guidance and Reflections on Recovery from Eating Disorders*, ed. Aimee Liu. Boston & London: Trumpeter, 2011, 13–15.

CHAPTER 11: FINDING COMPASSIONATE CARE

1   Academy for Eating Disorders, "World Wide Charter for Action on Eating Disorders 2005," http://www.aedweb.org/source/charter /documents/WWCharter4.pdf.

2   National Institute for Clinical Excellence, http://www.Nice .Org.Uk/Page.Aspx?O=101239.

3   Christine Peat, Kimberly Brownley, Nancy Berkman, and Cynthia Bulik, "Binge Eating Disorder Treatment: An Update." *Current Psychiatry Reviews* 11, no. 5 (2012): 33–39.

4   Aaron T. Beck, *Cognitive Therapy for Depression*. New York: Guilford Press, 1979.

5   Virginia McIntosh, Jennifer Jordan, Suzanne Luty, Frances Carter, Janice McKenzie, Cynthia Bulik, and Peter Joyce, "Specialist Supportive Clinical Management for Anorexia Nervosa." *International Journal of Eating Disorders* 39, no. 8 (2006): 625–32.

6   Gerald Klerman, Myrna Weissman, Bruce Rounsaville, and Eve Chevron, *Interpersonal Psychotherapy of Depression.* New York: Basic Books, 1984.

7   Christopher Fairburn, Rosemary Jones, Robert Peveler, Sally Carr, Ruth Solomon, Marianne O'Connor, Jenny Burton, and R. A. Hope, "Three Psychological Treatments for Bulimia Nervosa: A Comparative Trial." *Archives of General Psychiatry* 48, no. 5 (1991): 463–69.

8   Virginia McIntosh, Cynthia Bulik, Janice McKenzie, Suzanne Luty, and Jennifer Jordan, "Interpersonal Psychotherapy for Anorexia Nervosa." *International Journal of Eating Disorders* 27, no. 2 (2000): 125–39.

9   Denise Wilfley, Robinson Welch, Richard Stein, Emily Spurrell, Lisa Cohen, Brian Saelens, Jennifer Dounchis, Mary Anne Frank, Claire Wiseman, and Georg Matt, "A Randomized Comparison of Group Cognitive-Behavioral Therapy and Group Interpersonal Psychotherapy for the Treatment of Overweight Individuals with Binge-Eating Disorder." *Archives of General Psychiatry* 59, no. 8 (2002): 713–21.

10 Marsha Linehan, *Cognitive-Behavioral Treatment of Borderline Personality Disorder.* New York: Guilford Press, 1993.

11 William Miller and Stephen Rollnick, *Motivational Interviewing: Preparing People for Change.* Second Edition. New York: Guilford Press, 2002.

12 James Prochaska and Carlo DiClemente, "Stages and Processes of Self-Change of Smoking: Toward an Integrative Model of Change." *Journal of Consulting and Clinical Psychology* 51, no. 3 (1983): 390–95.

13 Steven Hayes, Jason Luoma, Frank Bond, Akihiko Masuda, and Jason Lillis, "Acceptance and Commitment Therapy: Model, Processes and Outcomes." *Behaviour Research and Therapy* 44, no. 1 (2006): 1–25.

14 Cynthia Bulik, Donald Baucom, Jennifer Kirby, and Emily Pisetsky, "Uniting Couples (in the Treatment of) Anorexia

Nervosa (UCAN)." *International Journal of Eating Disorders* 44, no. 1 (2011): 19–28.

15   American Psychiatric Association, "Practice Guideline for the Treatment of Patients with Eating Disorders, Third Edition," http://www.psychiatryonline.com/pracGuide/loadGuidelinePdf .aspx?file=EatingDisorders3ePG_04-28-06.

16   Ruth Striegel-Moore, Douglas Leslie, Stephen Petrill, Vicki Garvin, and Robert Rosenheck, "One-Year Use and Cost of Inpatient and Outpatient Services Among Female and Male Patients with an Eating Disorder: Evidence from National Database of Health Insurance Claims." *International Journal of Eating Disorders* 27, no. 4 (2000): 381–89.

17   Janice McKenzie and Peter Joyce, "Hospitalization for Anorexia Nervosa." *International Journal of Eating Disorders* 11, no. 3 (1992): 235–41.

18   Richard Matthias, "Care Provision for Patients with Eating Disorders in Europe: What Patients Get Treatment Where?" *European Eating Disorders Review* 13, no. 3 (2005): 159–68.

19   Stacey Solomon and Donald Kirby, "The Refeeding Syndrome: A Review." *Journal of Parenteral and Enteral Nutrition* 14, no. 1 (1990): 90–97.

20   Philip Mehler, Amy Winkelman, Debbi Andersen, and Jennifer Gaudiani, "Nutritional Rehabilitation: Practical Guidelines for Refeeding the Anorectic Patient." *Journal of Nutrition and Metabolism* 2010 (2010): 625782.

21   Kathleen Pike, B. Timothy Walsh, Kelly Vitousek, G. Terrence Wilson, and Joy Bauer, "Cognitive Behavior Therapy in the Posthospitalization Treatment of Anorexia Nervosa." *American Journal of Psychiatry* 160, no. 11 (2003): 2046–9.

22   Virginia McIntosh, Jennifer Jordan, Frances Carter, Sue Luty, Jan McKenzie, Cynthia Bulik, Christopher Frampton, and Peter Joyce, "Three Psychotherapies for Anorexia Nervosa: A Randomized Controlled Trial." *American Journal of Psychiatry* 162, no. 4 (2005): 741–7.

23   Cynthia Bulik et al., "Uniting Couples (in the Treatment of) Anorexia Nervosa."

24   Cynthia Bulik, Nancy Berkman, Kimberly Brownley, Jan Sedway, and Kathleen Lohr, "Anorexia Nervosa Treatment: A Systematic Review of Randomized Controlled Trials." *International Journal of Eating Disorders* 40, no. 4 (2007): 293–309.

25 Ibid.

26 Paul Appelbaum, "Commentary: Psychiatric Advance Directives at a Crossroads: When Can PADs Be Overridden?"
Journal of the American Academy of Psychiatry and the Law 34,
no. 3 (2006): 395–7.

27 Jacinta Tan, Anne Stewart, Raymond Fitzpatrick, and Tony
Hope, "Attitudes of Patients with Anorexia Nervosa to Compulsory Treatment and Coercion." *International Journal of Law
and Psychiatry* 33, no. 1 (2010): 13–9.

28 Ibid.

29 Jennifer Shapiro, Nancy Berkman, Kimberly Brownley, Jan
Sedway, Kathleen Lohr, and Cynthia Bulik, "Bulimia Nervosa
Treatment: A Systematic Review of Randomized Controlled
Trials." *International Journal of Eating Disorders* 40, no. 4
(2007): 321–36.

30 Fluoxetine Bulimia Nervosa Collaborative Study Group,
"Fluoxetine in the Treatment of Bulimia Nervosa: A Multi-
center, blacebo-controlled, Double-blind Trial." *Archives of
General Psychiatry* 49, no. 2 (1992): 139–47.

31 Kimberly Brownley, Nancy Berkman, Jan Sedway, Kathleen
Lohr, and Cynthia Bulik, "Binge Eating Disorder Treatment: A
Systematic Review of Randomized Controlled Trials." *Interna-
tional Journal of Eating Disorders* 40, no. 4 (2007): 337–48.

32 Linda Craighead and Heather Allen, "Appetite Awareness
Training: A Cognitive-Behavioral Intervention for Binge Eating."
Cognitive and Behavioral Practice 2, no. 2 (1995): 249–70.

33 Marsha Marcus and Michelle Levine, "Obese Patients with
Binge Eating Disorder." In *The Management of Eating Disor-
ders and Obesity*, ed. David Goldstein. New Jersey: Humana
Press, 2005, 143–60.

34 Virginia McIntosh, Jennifer Jordan, Janet Carter, Janet Latner,
and Alison Wallace, "Appetite Focused Cognitive-Behavioral
Therapy for Binge Eating." In *Self-Help Approaches for Obesity
and Eating Disorders: Research and Practice*, ed. Janet Latner
and G. Terrence Wilson. New York: Guilford Press, 2007,
325–46.

35 Kimberly Brownley et al., "Binge Eating Disorder Treatment:
A Systematic Review of Randomized Controlled Trials."

CHAPTER 12: IT'S NOT A LIFE SENTENCE, AND RECOVERY IS NOT SOLITARY CONFINEMENT

1   Anna Bardone-Cone, Megan Harney, Christine Maldonado, Melissa Lawson, D. Paul Robinson, Roma Smith, and Aneesh Tosh, "Defining Recovery from an Eating Disorder: Conceptualization, Validation, and Examination of Psychosocial Functioning and Psychiatric Comorbidity." *Behaviour Research and Therapy* 48, no. 3 (2010): 194–202.

2   Deborah Kasman, "When Is Medical Treatment Futile?" *Journal of General Internal Medicine* 19 (2004): 1053–56.

3   Amy Lopez, Joel Yager, and Robert Feinstein, "Medical Futility and Psychiatry: Palliative Care and Hospice Care as a Last Resort in the Treatment of Refractory Anorexia Nervosa." *International Journal of Eating Disorders* 43, no. 4 (2010): 372–7.

Index

Note: Italic page numbers refer to figures and tables.

A NOTE ON THE AUTHOR

Cynthia M. Bulik, Ph.D., FAED, is Distinguished Professor of Eating Disorders in the Department of Psychiatry in the School of Medicine at the University of North Carolina at Chapel Hill, where she is also professor of nutrition in the Gillings School of Global Public Health, and the director of the UNC Center of Excellence for Eating Disorders. Dr. Bulik, a clinical psychologist, has been conducting research and treating individuals with eating disorders for more than three decades. She developed treatment services for eating disorders both in New Zealand and in the United States. Her research has included treatment, laboratory, epidemiological, twin, and molecular genetic studies of eating disorders and body weight regulation. She has active research collaborations throughout the United States and in twenty countries around the world.

She is a recipient of the Eating Disorders Coalition Research Award, the Academy for Eating Disorders Leadership Award for Research, the Price Family National Eating Disorders Association Research Award, the Women's Leadership Council Faculty-to-Faculty Mentorship Award, and the Academy for Eating Disorders Meehan-Hartley Advocacy Award. She is a past president of the Academy for Eating Disorders, past vice president of the Eating Disorders Coalition, past associate editor of the *International Journal of Eating Disorders*, chair of the Scientific Advisory Council of the Binge Eating Disorder Association, and a member of the Scientific Advisory Committee of the Global Foundation for Eating Disorders. Dr. Bulik holds the first endowed professorship in eating disorders in the United States. Her academic life is balanced by being happily married with three children and being a gold medalist ice dancer.